YOGA
MEDITATION

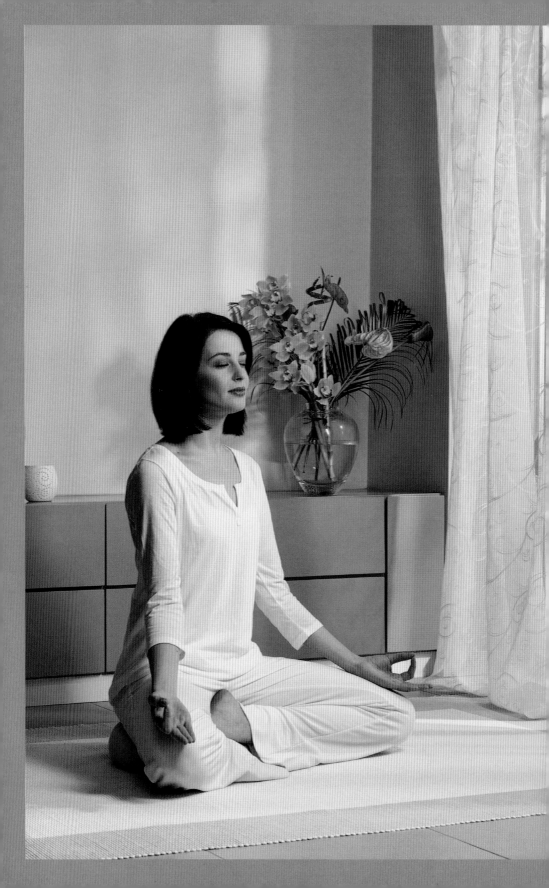

YOGA MEDITATION

STILL YOUR MIND AND AWAKEN YOUR INNER SPIRIT

STEPHEN STURGESS

WATKINS PUBLISHING

LONDON

Yoga Meditation
Stephen Sturgess

First published in the UK and USA in 2014 by
Watkins Publishing Limited
PO Box 883, Oxford OX1 9PL, UK

enquiries@watkinspublishing.co.uk

A member of Osprey Group

For enquiries in the USA and Canada:
Osprey Publishing
PO Box 3985, New York, NY 10185-3985
Tel: (001) 212 753 4402
Email: info@ospreypublishing.com

Managing Editor: Kelly Thompson
Senior Editor: Tania Ahsan
Managing Designer: Luana Gobbo
Picture Research: Cee Weston-Baker
Commissioned Artwork: Christiane Beauregard & Stephen Sturgess
Commissioned Photography: Jules Selmes
Make-up Artist: Justine Martin

A CIP record for this book is available from the British Library

ISBN: 978-1-78028-644-0
10 9 8 7 6 5 4 3 2 1

Typeset in Spectrum
Colour reproduction by PDQ, UK
Printed in China

Publisher's note: The information in this book is not intended as a substitute
for professional medical advice and treatment. If you are pregnant or are suffering
from any medical conditions or health problems, it is recommended that you consult
a medical professional before following any of the advice or practice suggested in this
book. Watkins Publishing Limited, or any other persons who have been involved
in working on this publication, cannot accept responsibility for any injuries or damage incurred as
a result of following the information, exercises or therapeutic techniques contained in this book.

Watkins Publishing is supporting the Woodland Trust, the UK's leading woodland
conservation charity, by funding tree-planting initiatives and woodland maintenance.

www.watkinspublishing.co.uk

This book is dedicated to my guru
Paramhansa Yogananda (1893–1952),
who brought the supreme technique
of Kriya Yoga meditation
to the West.

*"The wholehearted practice of meditation brings deep bliss.
This ever-new bliss is not born of desire; it manifests itself
by the magic command of your inner, intuitive-born calmness.
Manifest this serenity always."*

Paramhansa Yogananda

CONTENTS

What is True Happiness?

Knowingly or unknowingly, we are all seeking lasting happiness: a sense of calm, balance and completeness, true joy of total fulfilment, and freedom from suffering, pain and sorrow. Yet we can, at times, feel out of sync, lacking in joy, overwhelmed by life or have a sense that "something is missing".

We may have all the material comforts that life can give us — a house, a car, beautiful clothes, the latest technology, a good marriage or relationship, sex, family, friends, a successful career and good health — all the things that are believed by most people to bring happiness and security. But happiness may still elude us or feel all too fleeting — overshadowed by moments of worry, discontent or self-doubt. And what good is success in the external world if we have not found contentment, inner peace and true joy within?

Through not understanding the distinction between pleasure (an attribute of the senses) and happiness (an attribute of the mind), we often try to give our lives meaning and purpose by turning our minds outward. Hence we fill our time with external events, activities and objects — pursuits that can bring only transitory happiness.

If, on the other hand, we choose to turn our mind and senses inward through the practice of Yoga Meditation, as outlined in this book, we have the chance to transcend the everyday external limitations by which we are held back and be united with our true, innermost, joyful Self. This is known in Sanskrit as *Sat-Chit-Ananda*: ever-conscious, ever-existent, ever-new bliss. By encouraging the thinking mind to become still through meditation, we will allow the light of the true Self to start to shine from within.

As such, we can realize, and start to become established in, the awareness of what is often called in yogic terms our own divine nature, which recognizes the union of the individual self, or consciousness, with the Absolute, or Supreme, Consciousness. This allows us to experience a sense of underlying unity in the world and vibrant connectedness with everything.

When everything we do in life is an expression of this *inner* divine state of bliss, we regain our balance, freedom and joy, and experience true happiness every day. As such, it is a wise investment to devote some regular time to the Yoga Meditation practices in this book, as they will guide you on this path of emotional and spiritual discovery, calming your mind, heightening your clarity, enhancing your joy, awakening your inner spirit and allowing you to realize your fullest potential for creative thought and action.

What is Yoga Meditation?

To fully understand Yoga Meditation, it is useful firstly to gain an understanding of yoga in its true, broad sense rather than in the context of the limited physical, "on the mat" practice that has come to be associated with the term in the West.

The word *yoga* comes from the Sanskrit root *yuj*, which means "to yoke, join or unite". The ultimate meaning is the *union* between the individual self and the Universal Self. It is establishing *oneness* between the finite and the Infinite, between the inner being and the Supreme Being. So, as well as helping us to attain optimum health and a calm and peaceful mind, yoga can also lead us to self-realization and ultimately spiritual liberation and a sense of oneness with the Self.

*"Divine joy is like millions
of earthly joys crushed into one."*

Paramhansa Yogananda

THE YOGA OF MEDITATION

In this book the emphasis is on what is known as Raja Yoga – the yoga of meditation – which is principally concerned with the cultivation of the mind by learning to quieten or master its many fluctuations in order to experience deep stillness, joy and, ultimately, enlightenment. However, the pages that follow also contain physical purification practices for the body, breath and mind that derive from Hatha Yoga – the wider practice of yoga as defined in *Hatha Yoga Pradipika*. Such physical practices are also an essential part of Raja Yoga; Hatha and Raja Yoga are interdependent.

One way to think of the interaction between Hatha and Raja Yoga is that the physical practices of Hatha Yoga – *asana*, purification and *pranayama* practices (see chapters 4–6) – represent the cleaning of the temple windows (the physical body and mind) in order for the spiritual light of Raja Yoga – the meditation practices (see chapter 7) – to shine into the inner sanctum (the inner Self). After all, your physical body and mind are your primary tools for all spiritual practices. So without a strong, healthy body and mind, it is difficult to attain spiritual joy.

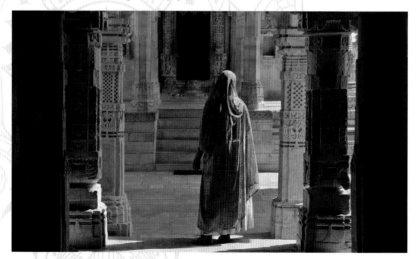

The teachings of Raja Yoga

Raja Yoga teachings can be traced back to around 200 BCE when they were systematized by a great sage called Patanjali, who formulated them into 196 aphorisms called the *Yoga Sutras*, quotes from which you will see scattered throughout this book. Some modern translations give the number of *sutras* as 195 due to the interpretation that one is an expansion of a previous *sutra*.

Patanjali's ancient guidelines give instruction on the actions he believed we need to take if we want to regain the experience of our true divine nature – from social and personal disciplines through yoga postures, breathing control and sense withdrawal to concentration and meditation techniques .

❋

Stilling the mind

Patanjali tells us in his *Yoga Sutras* that when the mind is still and turns within, we perceive the self in its true, divine, ever-joyful nature, free from any obstacles that were previously obscuring this:

"Yoga (the experience of unity) results from the neutralization of ego-feelings (vrittis) that produce desires, attachments, likes and dislikes."
Yoga Sutras 1:2

"Then the self abides in its own (eternal) true nature."
Yoga Sutras 1:3

"At other times when the self is not abiding in its own true nature, there arises false identification with the ego-feeling (vritti)."
Yoga Sutras 1:4

The Sanskrit word *vritti* means "whirlpool" and it is these swirling vortices of feeling arising from the ego – desires and attachments, likes and dislikes, feelings and memories – that cause restlessness of the mind. Yoga is simply the stilling of such feelings, and therefore of such movements, akin to waves gently stilling on the surface of a lake, bringing about a sense of calm.

KRIYA YOGA AND THE IMPORTANCE OF MEDITATION

In 1861, the ancient science of Raja Yoga, which had been lost for centuries, was revived as Kriya Yoga by the Himalayan yogi-master Mahavatar Babaji. In a succession of great masters, Babaji first taught Kriya to Lahiri Mahasaya (1828–1895), instructing him to teach it to sincere seekers of truth. Lahiri's spiritual descendent was Swami Sri Yukteswar Giri (1855–1936), who then instructed Paramhansa Yogananda (1893–1952), author of the spiritual classic *Autobiography of a Yogi* (1946).

In 1920, Paramhansa Yogananda was one of the first teachers to bring the teachings of yoga to the West. His Kriya Yoga teachings emphasized direct inner experience of the divine, which he called "self-realization". The idea of Kriya Yoga, which, along with Raja Yoga, is the basis for the invaluable Yoga Meditation practices in this book, is that it interiorizes the practitioner's concentration, reversing the outward-flowing life-energy (or *prana*) of the senses so that it moves inward and upward through the energy centres (or *chakras*; see pages 34-41) in the body, magnetizing the spine with energy and encouraging divine self-awareness.

So what is meditation?

It is important to consider for a moment what is really meant by the term "meditation" within the description of Raja, or Kriya, Yoga as the "yoga of meditation". Meditation is simply stilling the mind and liberating it from its restless emotions, thoughts, ego-feelings and desires so that a wonderful feeling of wholeness and being "at one" can be attained.

As human beings, we are a complex of body, mind and consciousness. In Western thought, mind and consciousness are sometimes used synonymously, which often causes misunderstanding to those who are new to Indian yoga philosophy. In yoga philosophy, the concepts of mind and consciousness indicate two different things: the mind exists only when there are thoughts. In the deep-sleep state no thoughts exist, and therefore there is no mind. You, on the other hand – that is to say your inner self – are consciousness itself, which is eternally present in the waking, dream and sleep states. It is only the light of the self or consciousness reflected on the mind that enables it to have powers of cognition and feeling. Yet we all too often fall into the trap of thinking that it is the mind itself that is the "knower" and the "light" in our everyday existence.

The practice of meditation allows you (your consciousness) to recognize the two entities as distinct through the act of observing your mind (your thoughts) just as you would observe an external object. In so doing, you come to recognize that you are not, in fact, the sum of your thoughts and that it is only once your thoughts quieten and your mind becomes still that you can recognize and feel at one with your true joyful self or consciousness, rather than continually associating with the ego, or external self, by which we are most often preoccupied.

❀

Everyday benefits of Yoga Meditation

As well as its underlying spiritual goal, Yoga Meditation brings a wide range of everyday benefits, enriching your life in all manner of ways. For example, it:

- gives you valuable time out for yourself
- helps to ease stress and anxiety
- increases your inner sense of calm and peace
- boosts your coping power in life
- strengthens your body from the inside out
- heightens concentration and clarity
- enhances powers of creativity
- allows you to feel more at one with yourself and the world
- encourages joy and happiness in every aspect of life.

THE JOURNEY WITHIN

It is my wish that this book, as well as enhancing how you feel within your own body – healthier and more vital – will also help to guide you on your inner journey to rediscover your true, peaceful, joyful nature – the divine and eternal Self within – which is the level at which you connect with supreme consciousness.

This journey – both health-enhancing and spiritual – can begin *here* and *now*. It will be your own personal journey – one that requires not only your awareness, willingness and effort but also sincerity, patience, self-discipline, perseverance and faith in yourself to succeed. Don't worry about how far from that state you currently feel: even a lotus needs to grow from within the mud toward sunlight.

True knowledge comes through direct experience so it is important to practise regularly, even if it is only for ten to 15 minutes a day. Although mornings or evenings are best, you can schedule your Yoga Meditation practice anytime. The only limitation is that you should not have eaten for at least two hours beforehand. If you suffer from asthma, diabetes, high blood pressure or heart problems, or are pregnant, you should not practise without expert guidance from a qualified teacher or medical practitioner.

Before you begin, it is important to understand that the practices that follow are not the goal in themselves. The art of Yoga Meditation is not merely doing techniques, for these are only vehicles to help you on your inner journey to attain the goal of yoga, or spiritual union. The techniques and practices will simply help you toward your goal and it is from this meditative state that true happiness will unfold from within. It takes time and dedication. This is why the practices on the pages that follow have been ordered in the way they have – so that you progress step by step on this journey to a calmer, happier, more fulfilled life. So relax and enjoy!

❁

How to use this book

Firstly, find a quiet and peaceful place to sit and read the introduction and chapters 1 and 2 to deepen your understanding of the yogic philosophy behind Yoga Meditation practices.

Next, read chapter 3 ("Preparing for Practice") so that you know the basics of how to sit and what factors to take into consideration during your practice.

Then, read through the techniques themselves – *asana* (see chapter 4), purification (see chapter 5), *pranayama* (see chapter 6) and meditation (see chapter 7) – so that you gain a sense of them all and will have an idea of how to do them when the time comes.

Finally, decide which of the Yoga Meditation routines from chapter 8, made up from the techniques throughout the book, you can do most comfortably on a regular basis, and enjoy integrating those practices into your life.

"On attaining the purity of the ultra-meditative state there is the pure flow of spiritual consciousness."
Yoga Sutras 1:47

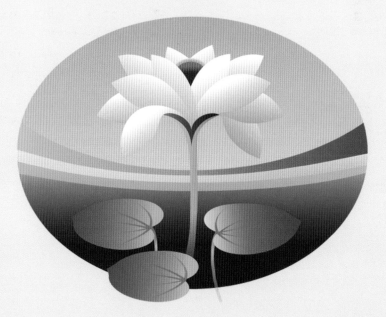

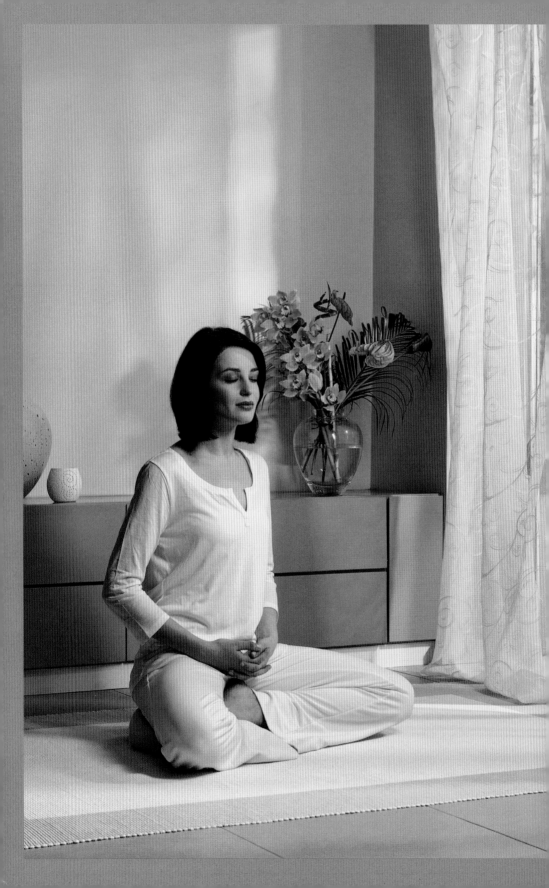

CHAPTER 1

THE EIGHT LIMBS OF YOGA

THE SUPREME PATH TO INNER FREEDOM AND JOY

Before you begin to explore the practical exercises and meditations in this book, it is useful to understand the concept of the "Eight Limbs of Yoga", called *ashtanga yoga* in Sanskrit (*ashta* means eight, *anga* means limb). These eight interdependent limbs, put forward by the sage Patanjali in his *Yoga Sutras* (c.200 BCE; see page 11), prepare us for the inward journey from our limited consciousness of outward identification with our body-mind, to a subtle, higher state in which we can feel more at one with ourselves and the universe. They provide the means for freedom from earthly "suffering" and the true awakening of our ever-joyful inner spirit.

The eight limbs, which we explore further in this chapter, are:

- *yama* – self-restraint
- *niyama* – fixed observances
- *asana* – yoga posture
- *pranayama* – regulation of life-force through the breath
- *pratyahara* – withdrawing the mind from the senses
- *dharana* – concentration
- *dhyana* – meditation
- *samadhi* – divine union

INTRODUCTION TO THE EIGHT LIMBS

The Eight Limbs of Yoga are methods of everyday purification advised by yoga sage Patanjali to help us on the path to a more fulfilled life. These include ethical principles and physical practices, as well as meditation techniques that prepare us for the final, higher stages of spiritual awakening.

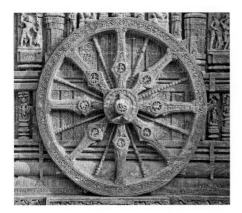

"From the sustained practice of the limbs of yoga, the impurities of the mind are destroyed, leading to the illumination of discriminative wisdom."

Yoga Sutras 2:28

YAMA — SELF-RESTRAINT

Yama is the first of the Eight Limbs of Yoga. The Sanskrit word *yama* means "restraint" — and in the context of the Eight Limbs, this means exercising restraint from actions, words and thoughts that may cause distress or harm either to ourselves or others. The five *yamas* are: non-violence; truthfulness; non-covetousness; conservation of vital energy; and non-attachment.

Ahimsa — non-violence
The root of all the *yamas* and *niyamas*, *ahimsa* means being kind and respectful to all living beings, including ourselves — not just in our actions but also in

our thoughts and words. For example, our speech should be honest and sincere, without gossiping or put-downs; our approach to Yoga Meditation practice should be gentle rather than laden with unrealistic expectations.

Satya – truthfulness

In yogic terms, to exaggerate, pretend, mislead, distort or lie to oneself or others, or to manipulate people or situations for our own selfish concerns, is against our true divine nature. Our essential nature is, in contrast, living in truthfulness. This not only means not lying to other people or ourselves, but also being true to our own feelings and beliefs.

Asteya – non-covetousness

To practise *asteya* means not to yearn or hanker after what does not belong to us. Desire, envy and greed keep us continually looking to the future for fulfilment, instead of realizing that perfection is attainable in the present, with what we are already lucky enough to have.

Brahmacarya – conservation of vital energy

The term *brahmacarya* ("walking in the presence of the divine") means wise use of our energy in all ways, as any kind of excess or over-indulgence, whether over-eating, over-sleeping, over-talking or even over-exercise, leads to dissipation of energy, which depletes our vitality.

Aparigraha – non-attachment

Practising *aparigraha* means not being overly attached to external objects or events, or the results that they might bring about. It means not being possessive about, or hoarding, objects, not trying to control other people and not holding on rigidly to thoughts, ideas and opinions. Even within Yoga Meditation practice, it's important to practise *aparigraha* by not being too fixed on desired results; instead, accept and move forward with what comes.

Niyama – Fixed Observances

The *niyamas* are the second of the Eight Limbs of Yoga and are just as important as the *yamas*, but are more about the connection with the individual than with the society around us. The five *niyamas* are: purity; contentment; self-discipline; self-study; and attunement to the supreme consciousness.

Sauca – purity

Practising *sauca* means ensuring cleanliness of both the body and the mind, which will enable us more readily to feel an enhanced state of inner calm and stillness. This involves simple physical measures such as washing each morning and before each Yoga Meditation practice, but it also implies freedom from all negative mental entanglements with objects, circumstances and thoughts. The practices in this book will help you to work toward ridding your mind of such entanglements.

Santosa – contentment

Practising *santosa* means being in a state of happiness and equanimity that does not depend upon any external conditions. This type of contentment is not conditioned by what we have or do not have as this will lead to a mind that cannot be satisfied permanently with anything. Instead we should aim to feel contented *within* ourselves. Regular practice of Yoga Meditation will naturally still the restless mind, enhancing your ability to remain calm and balanced in all situations.

Tapas – self-discipline

Tapas is energy that is concentrated with conscious willpower on a specific point, so that it releases power. For example, if you inhale deeply and tense your left arm with willpower, hold your breath and the tension for a few moments and then exhale and release the tension, you will feel the energy surge into your arm. Such energy is necessary for concentration of the mind.

The cultivation of self-discipline or *tapas* through the techniques in this book will enable you to overcome the egoistic nature of the mind and instead direct its power toward higher spiritual aims.

Svadhyaya – self-study

Together with *tapas* (below left) and *ishvara pranidhana* (below), *svadhyaya*, meaning self-study, works as a tool to weaken what are known in yogic terms as the five afflictions (*kleshas*): ignorance; egoism; attraction; repulsion; and fear of death. Self-study is not an intellectual process, but simply an *awareness* of the movements of the mind. It can be achieved through regular study of yoga scriptures such as the *Bhagavad Gita*, Patanjali's *Yoga Sutras* and the *Upanishads*, by chanting sacred mantras such as *Om* (see pages 132–3), and also by mindfully observing our ego-mind to gain insight into how it veils our understanding of our true self.

Ishvara pranidhana – attunement to the supreme consciousness

Ishvara pranidhana means the offering of our ego-self to the supreme consciousness. By remaining from moment to moment in the *awareness* and *presence* of this higher consciousness, we can transcend our daily sense of "I", "me" and "mine", thus inwardly realizing our own true, eternal nature and experiencing a deep sense of inner peace and unity.

"Supreme happiness is gained via contentment."
Yoga Sutras 2:42

ASANA – YOGA POSTURE

The most well-known and widely practised aspect of yoga in modern life is the notion of *asana*, meaning physical posture. However, Patanjali, who laid it out as the third of his Eight Limbs of Yoga, actually deals with the subject of *asana* in only three of his 196 *sutras*, referring only to seated postures such as *Sukhasana* (Easy Pose; see page 53), *Siddhasana* (Adept Pose; see page 55) and *Padmasana* (Lotus Pose; see page 56). This is because he is concerned with postures that bear a relationship to the overall purpose of yoga, which is concentration and meditation. And, according to him, postures that are steady, pleasant and comfortable will lend themselves to such concentration.

There are, however, many more varied yoga *asanas* that can be done for overall physical well-being (see chapter 4 for examples), as well as to energize and relax the body in preparation for meditation. In the *Hatha Yoga Pradipika* – a mid-14th-century treatise by Svatmarama Yogendra – we read: "*Asana* is the first stage of Hatha Yoga ... It gives steadiness, health and lightness of the body" (1:17).

Regular practice of the *asanas* in chapter 4 will help to purify and strengthen the body, open and balance the *chakras* (see pages 34–41), clear out blockages of the internal energy channels (*nadis*; see pages 42–5), and awaken the energy in the spine (*kundalini*; see pages 46–7) for the purpose of raising it to the higher centres in the brain during meditation.

"The posture should be steady and comfortable."
Yoga Sutras 2:46

PRANAYAMA –
REGULATION OF LIFE-FORCE THROUGH THE BREATH

Pranayama, the fourth of the Eight Limbs of Yoga, is defined in the *Yoga Sutras* as "regulation of the life-force through stilling the breath"(2:49). The Sanskrit word *pranayama* is formed from two words: *prana*, the energy or subtle life-force that permeates and sustains all life; and *ayama*, meaning "to regulate or extend". However, *prana* is not breath itself, and *pranayama* is not just regulating or controlling the breath; breath is simply the means of accessing the *prana*. *Pranayama* therefore involves regulating and harmonizing the life-force within the body – the energy that pervades the entire physical system and that acts as a medium between the body and the mind. By the process of *pranayama*, individual energy and consciousness are expanded into universal energy and consciousness.

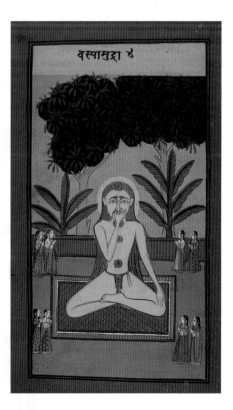

The *pranayama* practices in chapter 6 will help you not only to experience the pranic flow of life-energy in your body, but also to start to regulate it, and use it for energizing the body and calming the mind for meditation.

An 18th-century Indian miniature depicting a yogic breathing technique.

PRATYAHARA — WITHDRAWING THE MIND FROM THE SENSES

Pratyahara is the fifth of the Eight Limbs of Yoga, and relates to preparing the mind for concentration and meditation.

The Sanskrit word *pratyahara* is a combination of two words: *prati*, meaning "reverse direction"; and *ahar*, meaning "to remove or withdraw". *Pratyahara* therefore means "to retreat in the opposite direction": it is withdrawal of the mind from the five senses and their respective objects in the world – an interiorization of the mind.

Usually as we look at, listen to, smell, touch or taste something, our attention is drawn out of ourselves; whereas in *pratyahara* the attention is directed inward.

It is only through the practice of *asana* and *pranayama* that we can learn to turn the mind's attention inward in this way, being totally aware of where the impulse to breathe in and breathe out arises. By regularly doing these practices, we release ourselves from attachment to the duality of pleasure and pain, which causes us distress, and our minds can become still.

"By conscious interiorization of the mind, the senses function intelligently and in harmony without ego-mind interference. Therefore, one attains complete mastery over all the senses."

Yoga Sutras 2:55

DHARANA — CONCENTRATION

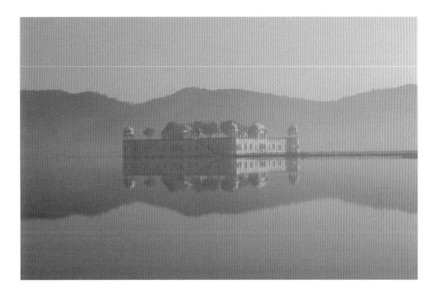

Dharana, or one-pointed concentration, is the sixth limb of Patanjali's Eight Limbs of Yoga, with the Sanskrit word *dharana* coming from the word *dhri*, "to hold firm".

The mind can be compared to a lake, with the thoughts and feelings that arise from the mind appearing as waves on the lake. We can see our reflection clearly in the waters only when the waves on the surface subside and become still. Similarly, we can realize our true inner self only when all the thought-waves and vortices of feelings (*vrittis*) in our mind are stilled through concentration on a single point, instead of being allowed to roam anywhere they please as an expression of the ego-self. *Tratak* (see page 113) and *Hong Sau* (see pages 122–5) are particularly effective methods for developing such concentration. And the more we can apply concentration in everyday life, the greater will be our success in meditation.

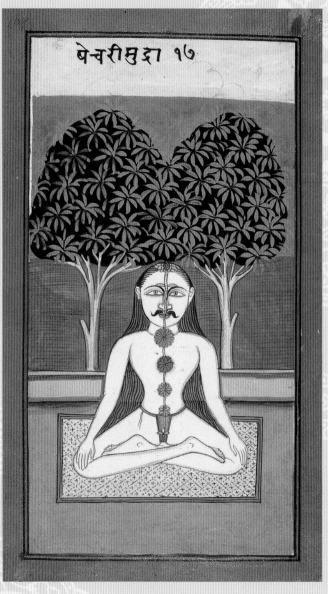

An 18th-century Indian painting showing a yogi in a
meditative asana, with the main chakras marked out.

"Meditation is the uninterrupted flow of attentive awareness
on the divine reality within."

Yoga Sutras 3:2

DHYANA – MEDITATION

Meditation, the seventh of the Eight Limbs, is liberation of the mind from all disturbing thoughts, emotional reactions and restless desires, and turning our attention inward to become aware of our own true blissful nature.

Meditation is not a technique per se, but a state of stillness and complete contentment in the present moment. All movement has ended with *dharana* (concentration), and in *dhyana* (meditation) we are at the inner source of our being, directly experiencing our true nature. All ideas about our identity as a separate and limited being are dispelled in the union of the individual consciousness and the Supreme Consciousness, and we come to realize that the infinite presence of the divine – *Sat-Chit-Ananda* (ever-conscious, ever-existing, ever-new bliss) – is always within us. The Yoga Meditation practices in the pages that follow will lead you on this path to *dhyana*, where you will experience deep calm and contentment.

SAMADHI – DIVINE UNION

The word *samadhi* comes from the Sanskrit terms *sam*, which means "perfect or complete", and *dhi*, which means "consciousness". It is the eighth of the Eight Limbs of Yoga. In the state of *samadhi* the mind is so totally absorbed in the divine Self that it is no longer aware of itself meditating. All distinctions between the person who is the subjective meditator, the act of meditation and the object of meditation merge into oneness.

The difference between meditation (*dhyana*) and *samadhi* is that in meditation there is an uninterrupted flow of attention toward the object of meditation, whereas in *samadhi* there is a complete dissolution of the subjective–objective duality of observer and observed. The meditator loses all sense of individuality (ego-consciousness), expansion of consciousness begins, and the mind merges into blissful oneness with the divine Self: the ultimate goal of all Yoga Meditation.

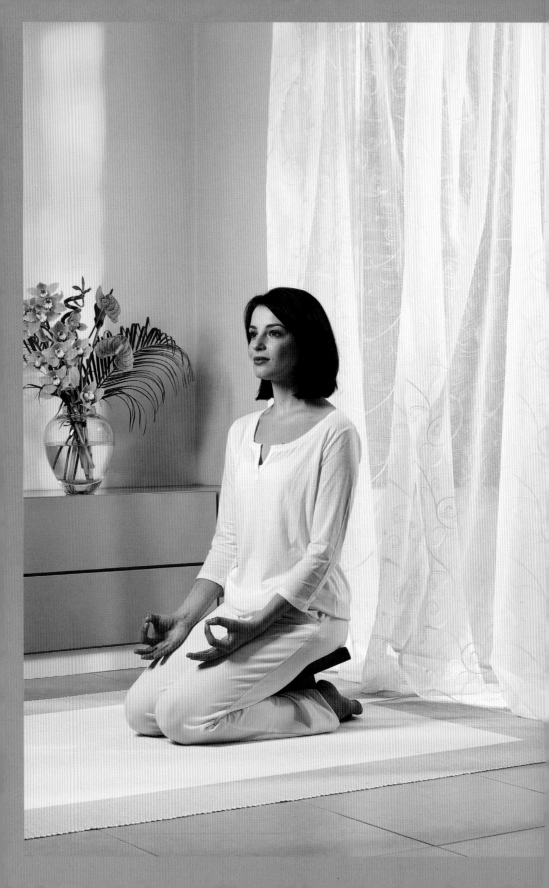

CHAPTER 2

THE INTERNAL ENERGY SYSTEM

SUBTLE BODIES, CHAKRAS, NADIS AND KUNDALINI

To understand the Yoga Meditation exercises in this book in all their aspects — physical, mental and spiritual — it is first helpful to have some knowledge and understanding of your subtle anatomy. The more you become aware of this internal energy system and can direct your own essential life-force efficiently, not only as you practise the exercises in this book but also as you go about your daily life, the more control you will enjoy over your own health and happiness.

In this chapter, we explore this energy system, including:

- the physical body, the two subtle bodies and their five sheaths (*koshas*) — the subtle bodies and sheaths sustain the physical body with energy, just as electricity powers light within a light bulb
- the *chakras* — the body's seven main energy centres serve as transformers to receive, assimilate and distribute the vital energy, or life-force, required for the body's systems to function
- the *nadis* — subtle energy channels running throughout the body transport the body's life-force, nourishing you with vitality
- *kundalini* — spiritual energy, or consciousness, which is symbolized as a coiled-up serpent living in a latent form at the base of the spine.

THE THREE BODIES AND FIVE SHEATHS

We are spiritual beings, immortal spirit-souls temporarily embodied in both material fields of energy (our physical body) and non-material fields of energy ("subtle bodies" that are invisible to the naked eye).

These subtle bodies interpenetrate and surround our physical body in two layers, known as the astral and the causal body.

The body in which our true self or soul (*atman* or *purusha*) resides can therefore be likened to a castle that has three layers of fortification:

- the physical body (*sthula sharira*) – the inner "wall", which is subject to the limits of time, space and gravity, and is destroyed upon death
- the astral body (*suksma sharira*) – the middle "wall", which is more durable
- the causal body (*karana sharira*) – the outer "wall", which is even more permanent, being carried through countless lifetimes.

There are also what is known as five "sheaths" (*koshas*), which are located within the three bodies. These are called sheaths because they are like coverings of the inner luminous self, just as a light bulb is covered by a lampshade. Although we experience the action of these sheaths as if they are a reality that make up our personality, they – along with the three bodies – have, in fact, no permanent reality. They are mere vehicles for the expression of the true self (*atman*), which lies distinct from them all and which we aim to find through the Yoga Meditation practices in this book.

While we need to keep each of the bodies and sheaths in optimal working order so that we remain healthy and vital, we should also aim to stop associating their actions with our limited sense of self, and instead start identifying with the true, divine self that lies beyond, where we will find deep inner peace and contentment.

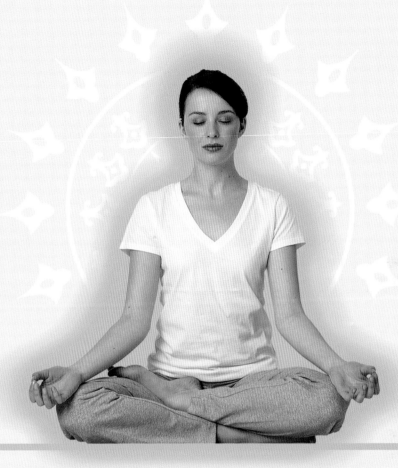

This image depicts the physical body (from which the golden glow of the soul, or atman, shines out) surrounded by the astral (yellow) and causal (green) bodies.

"The physical sheath is filled by the vital sheath,
the vital sheath by the mental sheath,
the mental sheath by the intelligent sheath,
and the intelligent sheath by the blissful sheath."

Taittiriya Upanishad

THE PHYSICAL BODY

The most concrete of the three bodies, the physical body is subject to birth, growth, disease, decay and death. The most effective way to keep this body healthy and vital is not only through a balanced diet and physical exercise such as running and swimming, but also through yoga postures (*asana*) to balance our energy, breathing techniques (*pranayama*) to clear the energy channels, and meditation to give rest to our mind and body.

The physical body has only one sheath, known as the *annamaya kosha*, or "food sheath", because of its dependence on life-force (*prana*) manifested in the forms of food, water and air. It sustains our physical existence.

THE ASTRAL BODY

The astral body – the invisible fortifying wall surrounding the physical body – is the home of our personality, our thoughts and our feelings; in short, all our non-physical personal attributes. This body could be described as the "conductor" of the physical body, as all our physical actions take place as a result of the astral body's energy (the physical body does not have the required energy of its own). The most effective way to energize and empower this body is through practising yoga *asana*, *pranayama*, mantra chanting (see page 112), self-enquiry and the study of yogic scriptures.

The astral body contains three sheaths: *pranamaya kosha*, *manomaya kosha* and *vijnanamaya kosha* (see below).

Pranamaya kosha – vital air sheath

This sheath supplies our life-energy, or *prana*, to the physical body, as well as controlling the organs of action (the hands, feet, tongue, genitals and anus), and governing how we react to the world.

Manomaya kosha – mind sheath

This is our mental and emotional layer, enabling us to experience our thoughts and feelings. Subtler than the food sheath and vital air sheath, the mind sheath communicates our thoughts and feelings to the physical body, which reacts accordingly. It also communicates our sensations of the external world, such as thirst or heat, to the intelligence sheath (see below) so that decisions can be taken on what to do about them. As such, it is a vital communicator. We can strengthen and purify this mind sheath by following certain *pranayama* and meditation practices.

Vijnanamaya kosha – intelligence sheath

This layer obtains knowledge through thought, experience and the senses. As such, it functions as the knower and the doer of the astral body, making decisions, choices and value-judgments. As well as being home to our intellect, this is where our ego resides – our strong sense of "I" and "my", which is what separates us from identifying with universal consciousness and finding our true, joyful inner self. To strive on a spiritual path, it is therefore important to aim to purify the ego and hone the intellect.

THE CAUSAL BODY

Even more subtle than the astral body, the causal body is composed of our deepest thoughts, desires, intentions and aspirations. It is the storehouse of our past impressions, the seed impressions that motivate our behaviour and create our karma. In the analogy of the three-walled castle, the causal body is the wall connecting us to the divine self. Although it gives light and energy to the astral body, its own vitality has a different abode, called the *anandamaya kosha* (bliss sheath). This is a body of light that reflects the blissfulness of the self, allowing us to experience true joy.

THE CHAKRAS

Chakra is a Sanskrit word meaning "wheel" or "revolving disc". Accordingly, *chakras* in the human body are thought to be wheels or revolving discs of subtle energy or life-force (*prana*) located along the midline of the astral body, known as the astral spine. They are confluences of consciousness and energy that store and distribute energy and information to the physical body, as well as storing our psychological tendencies, desires and habits.

The yoga tradition recognizes seven major *chakras* distributed along the midline of the body. These are located:

• at the base of the spine – *muladhara*
• in the genital area – *svadhisthana*

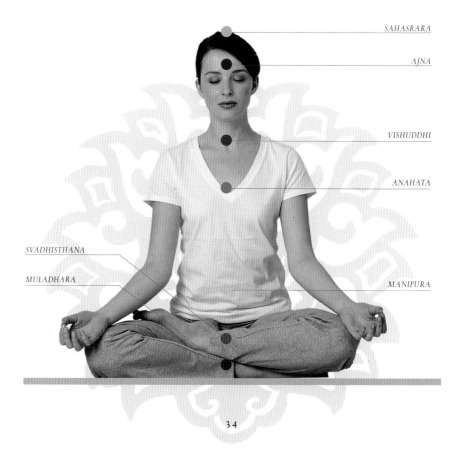

SAHASRARA

AJNA

VISHUDDHI

ANAHATA

SVADHISTHANA

MULADHARA

MANIPURA

- at the navel – *manipura*
- at chest or heart level – *anahata*
- at the throat – *vishuddhi*
- at the forehead – *ajna*
- above the crown of the head – *sahasrara*

It is essential for these *chakras* to be functioning well in order to store the maximum energy that can be used by the body at will. Just like, over a period of time, the battery of a car can become old and lose its capacity to "hold charge" if not well looked after, so too will your *chakras* become unable to adequately support the vital systems of the body if they are not sufficiently developed. Regular practice of the yoga exercises in the pages that follow, such as *asanas, pranayama* and chanting the *bija* mantras (see pages 118–9), will ensure their balanced development, and therefore boost energy levels and enhance overall health.

❀

Visual representation of the chakras

According to yogis, healers and psychics who are able actually to see human energy fields, *chakras* are colourful, fast-moving whirlpools, each one taking the form of a funnel-shaped structure, somewhat like a convolvulus flower. They are often symbolized by diagrams in the form of lotus flowers (*padmas*), each one with specific numbers of petals, colours, seed-syllable (*bija*) mantras and other symbols and deities within them. These images are visual representations of the *chakras*' energetic experiences (see chart on page 41) and can help meditators to achieve concentration of the mind. The colours of the *chakras* here do not tally with the Western New Age tradition but correspond to the yogic tantric tradition as elucidated by Swami Satyananda Saraswati (1923–2009).

COSMIC ENERGY

Ultimately, our bodies are nothing but energy. Our *chakras* act as dynamos of cosmic energy, allowing our subtle bodies to plug into the universal power source. They serve as transformers and regulators to receive, assimilate and distribute *prana* in the astral body, which then distributes it to the spinal nerve plexuses, where it is, in turn, transferred to the blood and organs of the physical body.

The *prana* enters the body at the base of the brain (an area known as the medulla oblongata) and flows to the higher brain centres. It then filters downward through the six major *chakras* below that, starting at *ajna chakra* and working its way down to *muladhara chakra*; *sahasrara*, the main generator of the energies that power these six *chakras,* is located at the crown, above the medulla oblongata, and operates on a higher plane of consciousness.

As this energy spirals down through each *chakra,* it becomes increasingly dense, until it forms what are known as the five great elements (*panchamahabhuta*). These are essential "states" of matter, not to be confused with the periodic elements of modern chemistry, and they represent the stages of creation from spirit to matter.

- From the unmanifested state of universal consciousness came the subtle, primal sound vibration *Om*. From the subtle vibration of *Om* came the ether or space element – associated with *vishuddhi chakra*.
- The light and expansive movements of the ether element created the air element – associated with *anahata chakra*.
- The movement of air created friction, which generated heat particles forming intense light, from which the fire element was created – associated with *manipura chakra*.
- The heat of the fire liquefied certain ethereal elements that formed the water element – associated with *svadhisthana chakra*.
- Finally, the water solidified to form the earth element – associated with *muladhara chakra*.

Thus, the five building blocks of matter — ether, air, fire, water and earth — came into existence. These five elements, which are present in all matter, also exist within each of us. For example, in our body, the source of fire is metabolism — it activates our digestion and also activates our eyes to see light. The difference between the different elements in our body lies in their vibratory wavelength frequencies. The lower *chakras*, connected with basic survival and groundedness, vibrate at a denser frequency than the higher *chakras*, associated with spiritual enlightenment.

The underlying aim of the Yoga Meditation practices in this book is a reversal of the soul's descent into matter — back to divine oneness in pure consciousness, as it is only once this has been achieved that we can experience our true inner stillness and bliss. When your mind is calm and still, you become aware of your true identity, of the spiritual being within yourself who is beyond the forces of the body, mind and senses. Yoga Meditation is an effort to perceive this presence of cosmic energy and pure consciousness.

"The conscious cosmic energy first enters through the medulla oblongata (in the brain stem) and remains concentrated in the brain as the thousand-petalled lotus. Then it descends into the body through the spinal cord and sympathetic nervous system."

Paramhansa Yogananda

THE SEVEN CHAKRAS

Below is an overview of each *chakra*, the nature of its energy, and how that energy governs a certain aspect of our being, as well as insight into how each *chakra* fits into the Yoga Meditation journey in terms of raising our consciousness to a higher realm in our quest to discover our true, joyful inner self.

Muladhara – root chakra

Also referred to as the "base" chakra, *muladhara chakra* — located between the origin of the reproductive organ and the anus — is the foundation of our personality. When fully functioning, this *chakra* gives us a sense of groundedness and deep-seated security in life. It is also where *kundalini* energy (see pages 46–7) resides and is therefore the basis from which the possibility of higher realization arises: the upward journey of *kundalini* energy to *sahasrara chakra*, at the crown of the head, starts here, once it has been awakened through Yoga Meditation practices.

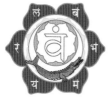

Svadhisthana – sacral chakra

Next on the journey up toward spiritual awakening is the fluid and adaptive *svadhisthana chakra* — located in the sacral region of the spine at the level of the coccyx (tailbone) — from where we can start to express ourselves creatively and sensually. When functioning well, this *chakra* gives us the ability to go with the flow and enjoy all that life has to offer.

The Sanskrit word *sva* means "one's own" and *adhisthana* means "dwelling place", so *svadhisthana* means "one's own dwelling place". It has been suggested by some yogis that this refers to a distant time when the seat of *kundalini* lay dormant within *svadhisthana chakra*, but for some reason *kundalini* has since come to rest in *muladhara chakra*.

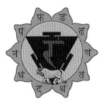

Manipura – navel chakra

Next we come to *manipura chakra*, which is said to radiate its fiery energy like a bright sun. It is located at the level of the navel in the astral spine. *Manipura* is a very important centre because it is the centre of willpower, energy, vitality and achievement. It generates and distributes *prana* throughout the whole body, and controls our energy, balance and strength. So when it is in balance, we will feel strong, self-confident, empowered and vibrant.

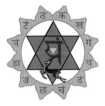

Anahata – heart chakra

Next, we ascend to *anahata chakra*. Also called the heart *chakra* due to its location, this functions as a bridge between the three lower *chakras* – related to the world of body, mind and senses and associated with survival and security (*muladhara chakra*), sensuality and sex (*svadhisthana chakra*), and a sense of identity and personal power (*manipura chakra*) – and the three higher *chakras*, associated with a higher and more evolved consciousness. The expansiveness of love and compassion in *anahata* draws us upward into the higher realms of consciousness. When this *chakra* is functioning well, we will feel great love and compassion in our life.

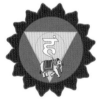

Vishuddhi – throat chakra

Located directly behind the base of the throat is *vishuddhi chakra*. The term *vishuddhi* is derived from the Sanskrit words *visha*, meaning "impurity", and *shuddhi*, meaning "to purify". It is our hub of communication, creativity, self-expression, non-attachment, and learning to accept and receive. When this *chakra* is balanced and open, our powers of communication and creativity become fully awakened. When *kundalini* energy reaches *vishuddhi*, we feel contentment, clarity of mind, a sense of understanding and non-attachment.

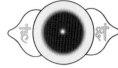

Ajna – third eye chakra

The Sanskrit word *ajna* literally means "to command", "to obey" or "to know". As such, this *chakra* – which is located on the forehead, between our eyebrows – is the command centre that guides the other *chakras*. Forming the boundary between human and divine consciousness, it represents a higher level of awareness and is considered the centre of extrasensory perception, intuition, clarity and wisdom.

Ajna chakra has two poles: a positive and a negative. The positive pole is the "spiritual eye", which is located midway between the eyebrows, while the negative pole is at the medulla oblongata, which is located in the brain stem at the base of the skull and is the seat of the ego.

Ajna chakra is the meeting point of the three main energetic channels (the *ida*, *pingala* and *sushumna nadis*; see pages 42–5). When *kundalini* energy reaches this *chakra*, our awareness becomes concentrated and our ego-self is transcended. It is here that we experience realization of our true divine self.

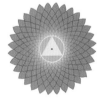

Sahasrara – crown chakra

Also called *niralambapuri*, meaning "dwelling place without support", and *Brahmarandhra*, "the door of God", *sahasrara chakra* is the culmination of our ascent of the astral spine – after achieving self-realization at *ajna*, we achieve liberation at *sahasrara*. To reach this point, first we need to open, balance and energize the six chakras below it through deep meditation.

Chakra Qualities and Elements

	LOCATION	POSITIVE QUALITIES	NEGATIVE QUALITIES	ELEMENT
SAHASRARA	crown of head	beyond all duality, bliss		beyond all elements
AJNA	centre of brain	selfless service, strong willpower, divine surrender	pride, excess intellect, strong sense of "I, me, mine"	*mahat*, i.e. mind, ego and intellect
VISHUDDHI	throat	expansiveness, sense of calm, silence	restlessness, boredom	ether
ANAHATA	heart	devotion, unconditional love, compassion	attachment, anger, rage, hatred	air
MANIPURA	navel	enthusiasm, confidence, effective leadership	misuse of power, ruthlessness	fire
SVADHISTHANA	sacrum	openness, willingness, intuition, creativity	indecision, vagueness	water
MULADHARA	perineum	courage, loyalty, steadfastness, perseverance	stubbornness, prejudice, intolerance	earth

THE NADIS

Within each of us lies a vast matrix of fine energetic channels called *nadis* (*nadi* literally means "flow" or "current"), which distribute our *prana*, or vital life-force throughout the body. These can be thought of as a network of interconnected rivers, streams and tributaries carrying energy to wherever it is needed. Indeed, the three main *nadis* (see below) are often symbolized by three of India's great rivers: the *ida* by the Ganges, the *pingala* by the Yamuna, and the *sushumna* by the mythical Saraswati.

The source of the *nadis* is an egg-shaped centre of nerves called the *kanda*, which is located just above our lowest energy centre, *muladhara chakra* (see page 38). From here some 72,000 *nadis* are said to radiate out to form the entire subtle circuitry of the astral body.

Of the thousands of nadis, three stand out as the most important. These, as mentioned above, are:

- the *sushumna* – the central channel, which corresponds in position to both the physical and astral spine
- the *ida* – which begins on the left side of the *sushumna*
- the *pingala* – which begins on the right side of the *sushumna*.

The *sushumna* is criss-crossed in a helix by the *ida* and *pingala*, and the three channels converge at certain locations along the spine, into the whirling vortices that are the *chakras* (see page 45).

It is useful to know a little more about each of the three main *nadis* so that you have an idea of what is happening to you energetically not only as you go about your daily life, but also as you do the Yoga Meditation practices on the pages that follow.

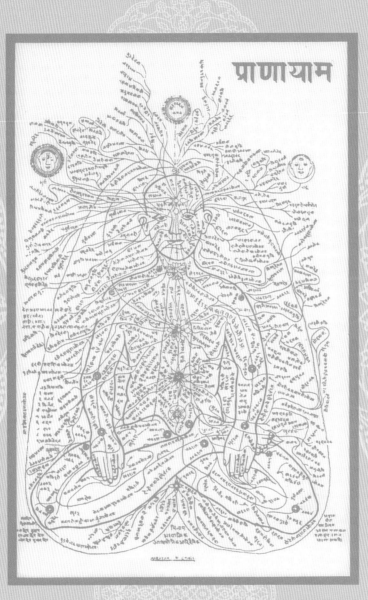

There is a matrix of thousands of energetic channels, known as nadis,
which comprise the subtle circuitry of the astral body.

THE SUSHUMNA

The *sushumna nadi* (meaning "most gracious channel") runs up the centre of the astral spine, which corresponds to the spinal cord in the physical body. This means that it passes through all the *chakras* in succession, from the base (*muladhara*) to the crown (*sahasrara*). While the *ida* and *pingala nadis* control our normal consciousness and are constantly active, even during sleep, the *sushumna nadi* is fully active only in people who are regularly engaged in spiritual practices such as Yoga Meditation. This is because it is only via such practices that balance can be achieved between *ida* and *pingala* energies, which, in turn, awakens the spiritual power known as *kundalini* (see pages 46–7), at the base of the spine, and sends it on its ascent along the *sushumna*. Also known as the *Brahma nadi* ("path to God"), the *sushumna* therefore provides the path to our spiritual awakening at *sahasrara chakra*: the place at which we can realize our true, joyful inner spirit and find the sense of inner calm for which we all search.

THE IDA AND THE PINGALA

The *ida* and *pingala nadis* function alternately in the body, not simultaneously. This can be seen in the nostrils as we breathe. Generally, breath is flowing freely through one nostril while the other is blocked. This natural alternation occurs approximately every two hours.

When the left nostril is open, the *ida nadi* is flowing, the right hemisphere of the brain is active, the mind is introverted and creative, and the parasympathetic nervous system is active – responsible for resting the body when required.

When the right nostril is open, the *pingala nadi* is flowing, the left hemisphere of the brain is active, the mind is extroverted and logical, and the sympathetic nervous system is more active – responsible for stimulating urgent action when required.

Ida

The *ida* channel transports mental energy (*chitta shakti*) throughout the body and therefore controls all our psychological processes. The Sanskrit word *ida* actually means "comfort", tying in with the notion of this channel being connected to the parasympathetic nervous system, which "comforts" and rests the body when it needs it. The *ida* is therefore associated with feminine, lunar energy, possessing cooling qualities.

Pingala

Conversely, the right-hand *pingala* channel transports our vital life-force (*prana*) throughout the body and therefore controls all our *physiological* processes. The Sanskrit word *pingala* means "tawny-red", which symbolizes this channel's association with the stimulating energy of the sun and links it to the function of the sympathetic nervous system, which is there to stimulate action when required. The *pingala* is therefore linked with masculine, solar energy, possessing heating qualities.

The ida and the pingala nadis criss-cross the central sushumna nadi, intersecting at chakras along the way.

KUNDALINI

Kundalini is the potential spiritual energy, or consciousness, that lies dormant at the base of the spine in the causal body (see page 33) of all beings. In reality, *kundalini* has no form, but as our mind requires a particular image on which to concentrate, *kundalini* has, in yogic theory, symbolically taken the form of a coiled serpent lying at the base of the spine (*kundalini* is derived from the Sanskrit term *kundal*, which means "coiled").

Another association with the term *kundalini* is the Sanskrit word *kunda*, which means "cavity" and refers to the concave space in which the brain, resembling a coiled, sleeping serpent, nestles.

Kundalini takes two forms:

- pranic energy (*prana shakti*), which is the cause of all our actions
- spiritual energy or consciousness (*caitanya shakti*), which gives rise to our knowledge and wisdom.

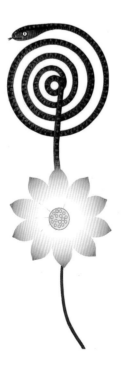

When dedicated Yoga Meditation practice brings about balance between the upward movement of energy in the *ida* (accompanied by inhalation) and the downward movement of energy in the *pingala* (accompanied by exhalation), *kundalini* is activated from its dormant state in *muladhara chakra*. Both these currents of energy then move upward in the central channel of the *sushumna*, where they are activated in the brain, creating a sense of inner calm and divine joy as part of our spiritual awakening.

As the *kundalini* makes this spiritual ascent from *muladhara chakra* (root *chakra*) towards the *sahasrara chakra* (the seat of consciousness, at the crown of the head), it activates all the *chakras* in succession, causing layer after layer of the mind to become opened until the yogi experiences a sense of awakening, freedom, inner calm, bliss and, ultimately, a sense of unity with the world.

When, on the other hand, *kundalini* remains dormant at the base of the spine, and the energy flow in the spine is downward, toward the three lower *chakras* of worldly consciousness – which it is likely to be in people who are not regularly following any kind of spiritual practice – a person is likely to feel a lack of inner calm, joy and contentment due to the duality they experience between themselves and the world around them.

Alternatively, for people who have just started practising Yoga Meditation or who don't yet do it regularly, there may only be a mild, or temporary, spiritual awakening – for example, in the lower three *chakras*. This would make them feel that there must be more to life than just eating, sleeping and sensual gratification (which operate in the three lower *chakras*). They are likely to be more aware that they are not just the body, mind and senses, but rather a spiritual being merely expressing themselves through these instruments.

However, regular practice of the *pranayama* exercises in chapter 6 will both purify and balance the *nadis*, increasing the chances of your experiencing the full potential and bliss of awakened *kundalini*.

"The kundalini, in its latent form, is coiled like a serpent.
One who causes that shakti to move (from the muladhara upward)
will attain liberation."

Hatha Yoga Pradipika 3:108

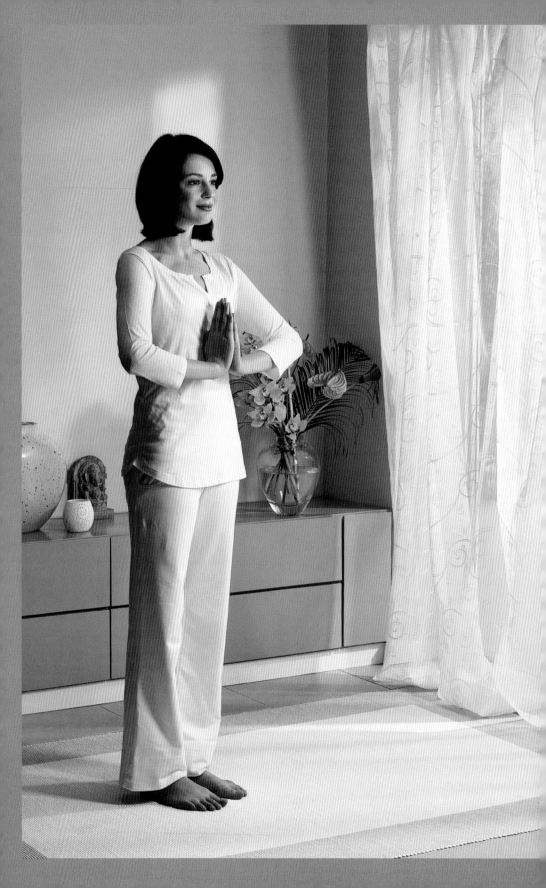

CHAPTER 3

PREPARING FOR PRACTICE

THE FUNDAMENTAL TOOLS YOU WILL NEED

The aim of this chapter is to set you up with the information you will need in order to work comfortably and effectively through the exercises and meditation practices in the rest of the book.

Firstly, you will discover the value of setting a regular time and space for your Yoga Meditation, as well as the importance of maintaining the right mental attitude to work toward your goals.

Secondly, you will discover the value of being able to sit still in a comfortable and steady posture, so that you can remain relaxed and alert for a considerable length of time without distraction. To achieve this effect, you will be offered instruction on a range of different seated postures, from which you can choose when it comes to doing your own meditation.

And finally you will be given an explanation of a range of yogic hand gestures called *mudras*, and internal yogic body "seals" or "locks" called *bandhas*. These can help to increase the power of your energy, retaining it and directing it upward through the energy centres (*chakras*), which will deepen your Yoga Meditation practice.

PRELIMINARIES FOR PRACTICE

To reap the greatest benefits from the Yoga Meditation techniques in this book, first set the intention to *want* to get in touch with your deep, innermost joyful self. Then, make a genuine commitment to yourself to work steadily toward that goal. Below are several other critical factors to take into account.

Timing

Traditionally, yogis meditate around sunrise and sunset, as the mind naturally becomes more calm and serene at these times. This is optimal. However, if these times are difficult for you, simply decide on the times that best suit *you* and commit yourself to setting these aside each day.

Regularity

The key to success in meditation is to develop and maintain a *regular* practice – daily if possible (as often as possible if not), and at the same time each day, for approximately the same length of time. This way, your body and mind will get accustomed to the regularity, and it will be much easier to get into the right state of mind for meditation each day.

Right attitude

The journey to a calmer, more contented self is a long, gradual process, so you will need to be patient and persevere. There is no instant success in spiritual life. It's therefore important to keep your Yoga Meditation practice high on your list of daily priorities and to practise with enthusiasm each time. Only by doing this will you feel like you are making progress and start to realize that the benefits of meditation – calmness, contentment and increased energy levels – are actually your natural state of being; you have just temporarily lost touch with it. You should also keep in mind the *yamas* and *niyamas* outlined on pages 18–21.

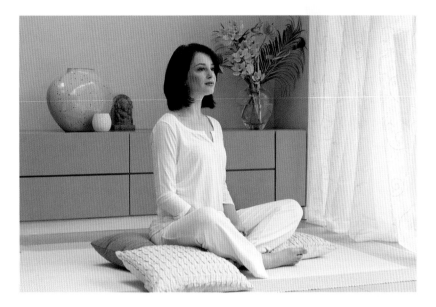

Preparing your space

Do your Yoga Meditation practice in a clean, tidy, quiet place, where you are unlikely to be disturbed. For comfort, it's best to wear loose, unrestrictive clothing, with all belts, jewellery, glasses and shoes removed. If you want to create a mood suitable for meditation, feel free to burn an incense stick or light a candle somewhere safe. As for props, there's just a couple of things you will need: a yoga mat on which to practise your *asanas* and a firm cushion on which to sit while you meditate. By sitting in the same place each time, you will build an aura of purity and peace there.

Preparing your body

The stomach should be at least half empty when you practise Yoga Meditation, so always allow at least two hours after a meal before you start. Do not practise if you are feeling ill or tired, or if you are feeling very upset, as the mind will not be able to concentrate.

THE ART OF SITTING
FOR MEDITATION

For effective Yoga Meditation practice, the body needs to be seated in a comfortable and steady posture – a position in which the natural curves of the spine can be maintained. The head, neck and spine should be upright and in alignment to allow energy to flow freely up to the higher *chakras*. You should be seated in such a way that you are able to remain still in that position for a significant amount of time. When such a position can be held without effort, the body can become relaxed, the breath steady and quiet, and the focused mind will be able to enter a deep state of stillness.

The pages that follow contain a range of seated positions to choose from, depending not only on your overall flexibility and comfort levels but also on what feels appropriate on any given day. The only way to discover which one is best for you is to try all of them, but be sure to go easy on yourself – never force a position and slowly alter your position if at any point you experience pain.

❀

Sitting on a chair

If you are unable to sit comfortably on the floor, the best option is to sit on an upright chair that has no armrests. Sit forward slightly to avoid leaning against the back rest. Keep your spine upright and place your feet hip-width apart on the ground. If they do not reach the floor, support them with folded blankets. Your lower legs should be perpendicular to the floor and your hips slightly higher than your knees.

Easy Pose – *Sukhasana*

❀

As the English name implies, this is the "easiest" or gentlest of the seated meditation postures, involving simply sitting cross-legged on the floor. However, it is not suitable for everyone so try it and see how you feel.

1 Sit on the floor on the edge of a firm cushion or folded blanket, bend in both legs and cross one leg on top of the other in front of you, so that your knees relax down to the sides. If you are more experienced, you may not need a cushion.

2 Ensure the cushion or blanket is an appropriate height to make the posture comfortable for you. Ideally, your knees should be slightly lower than your hips, or at least at the same level. This allows your thighs to relax downward, reducing tension in the hips and freeing the spine to lengthen upward.

3 Sit upright with the weight of your body in the front edges of your sitting bones. Align the upper body directly over the base of the spine. Lengthen the spine, open your chest and draw your shoulders back.

4 Rest your hands, palms upward, in *Chin Mudra* (see page 58) on your knees or thighs, depending on your preference.

Thunderbolt Pose – *Vajrasana*

❀

This kneeling meditation pose is a slight variation on the standard sitting theme and is one that is regularly used by Muslims and Zen Buddhists in prayer and meditation. Kneeling in *Vajrasana* calms and harmonizes the body and mind, activates *prana* in the *sushumna nadi* and redirects sexual energy to the brain for spiritual purposes.

1　Kneel on a yoga mat or cushion with your knees together and sit your buttocks on your heels.

2　Bring your big toes together and separate your heels, so that your buttocks are seated on the inside surface of your feet with your heels touching the sides of your hips.

3　Keep your body upright, with your head, neck and spine naturally aligned and relaxed.

4　Rest your hands, palms upward, in *Chin Mudra* (see page 58) on your knees or thighs.

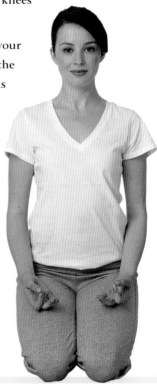

CAUTION: Be particularly careful with this pose if you have any issues with your knees, and, if you experience any pain in your thighs, separate your knees slightly.

Adept Pose – *Siddhasana*

❀

The Sanskrit term *siddha* means "perfected" or "accomplished". As such, it is no great surprise that *Siddhasana* is considered an ideal meditation posture among adept yogis. This is because it quietens the mind, has a balancing effect on the *nadis* and activates the spiritual energy of the *chakras* due to the pressure applied by the position of the feet.

1 Sit on the floor on the edge of a firm cushion or folded blanket. If you are more experienced, you may not need a cushion or blanket. Bend your left leg and place the sole of your foot flat against your inner right thigh with your heel pressing against the groin, so that you are essentially sitting on your left heel.

2 Then bend your right leg and place the right foot directly in front of the left foot so that the ankle bones are touching. Your left heel might press the pubic bone, directly above the genitals.

3 As an alternative, push the outer edge of the left foot and the toes between the right calf and thigh muscles. Grasp the right toes and pull them up in between the left calf and thigh.

4 Rest your hands, palms upward, on your knees in *Chin Mudra* (see page 58).

Lotus Pose – *Padmasana*

❈

Padmasana, meaning "lotus seat", is the classic sitting pose for Yoga Meditation, in which the feet are placed on opposing thighs. As the legs are in a bound position, the blood flow to them is reduced, resulting in an increase of blood flow to the brain, which purifies the nervous system. This posture has a balancing influence on all the *chakras* and brings an incomparable feeling of calm to the mind.

1 Sit on the floor with your legs extended in front of you. Then, slowly and carefully bend in your right leg, holding your right foot with both of your hands.

2 Turn the foot around so that the sole is facing you and place the instep up high on your left thigh as you lower your right knee to the floor. Your right heel should be close to your pubic bone.

3 Then bend in your left leg and, holding your left foot with your hands, place the instep up high on your right thigh. Find a point of comfort here.

4 Rest your hands, palms facing upward, on your knees in *Chin Mudra* (see page 58).

Adapted Lotus with Support

❀

This adapted version of the difficult-to-accomplish Lotus Pose is a good alternative for anyone who finds the seated floor positions uncomfortable for any reason (for example, stiff knees or sore back) but who doesn't want to sit on a chair. You will need five or six soft blankets to try it.

1 Sit on four or five folded blankets, with your back upright against a wall if your back muscles don't feel up to supporting themselves.

2 Bend your legs, crossing one over the other so that your shins contact each other, and each foot rests on the floor under the opposite knee.

3 Adjust the height of your knees until the kneecaps are pointing directly outward.

4 Place a long, rolled blanket around the front of your shins and over the tops of both feet and tuck it in firmly so that it supports your legs.

5 Tilt your pelvis forward and sit upright. Roll the tops of your shoulders back and lean your head gently against the wall.

6 With your head, neck and spine in alignment, keep your chest lifted and relax your abdomen and diaphragm muscles as you breathe slowly and rhythmically.

7 Rest your hands, palms facing upward, on your thighs, in *Chin Mudra* (see page 58).

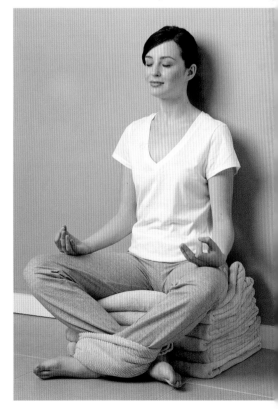

MUDRAS

A useful tool to get acquainted with are yogic gestures called *mudras*; *mudra* is a Sanskrit word meaning "gesture" or "attitude". *Mudras* can be applied to the hands, head or body, with the intention of awakening the *prana* to bring deepened awareness and concentration. Here we look at hand *mudras*. However, you will come across a range of other *mudras* in the exercises on the pages that follow, which are specific techniques relevant to specific practices; each is explained in its own section.

Your hands are essentially an energy map of consciousness. Each finger contains numerous nerve terminals and represents a certain quality. When fingers and parts of the palms connect in a particular hand *mudra*, it's like flicking a switch that activates *prana* along specific *nadis* in the hands, into the body, through the *chakras* and to the brain. This loop of energy between the brain and the hand *mudra* means that the pranic energy is unable to escape from the body and is therefore heightened, strengthening the body–mind connection. The four *mudras* that follow are the key hand positions for Yoga Meditation, and can be used interchangeably depending on the effect you would like to achieve.

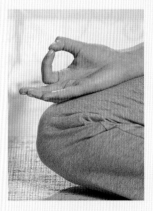

Chin Mudra – Gesture of Consciousness

Rest your hands, palms up, on your knees or thighs, and lightly join the tips of your thumbs and index fingers. Extend the other fingers. The word *chin* comes from the Sanskrit word *chit* or *chitta* meaning "consciousness". The closed circuit of the index finger and thumb symbolizes the union of the individual soul with supreme consciousness, making you feel calm and connected.

Jnana Mudra – Gesture of Wisdom

Rest your hands, palms down, on your knees or thighs, and lightly join the tips of your thumbs and index fingers. Relax the other fingers. *Jnana* (pronounced "gyana") *Mudra* gives stability, balances the five vital elements of the body, inspires creativity, develops the intellect, sharpens memory and increases concentration.

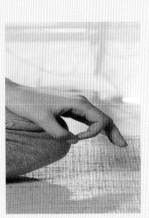

Bhairava Mudra – Gesture of Bliss

Rest your hands, palms upward, in your lap. Place the left hand on the right one, so that you cradle the back of your left hand in your right palm. Bring the tips of your thumbs together. The two hands represent the *ida* (left *nadi*) and *pingala* (right *nadi*), so their union symbolizes drawing the two energies together in the *sushumna* (central *nadi*), which has a deeply calming effect.

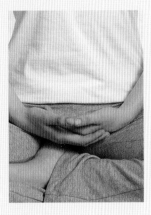

Clasped–hands *Mudra* – Gesture of Unity

Rest your hands, palms upward, in your lap. Interlock your fingers so that the fingers of each hand lie against the back of the opposite hand. Rest one thumb on top of the other. This is a symbol of mind and body in harmonious unity; the mind symbolized by the left thumb and the body by the right. Use this *mudra* to go deeper into meditative calm.

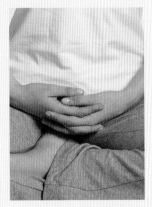

BANDHAS

Another useful yogic tool for Yoga Meditation is an understanding of internal energetic seals or locks known as *bandhas*. The Sanskrit word *bandha* means "to lock" or "to hold".

When a *bandha* is practised by applying a physical contraction to a specific body part, the energy flow is temporarily blocked, and controlled. When the *bandha* is released, the energy flows more strongly in that area, with increased pressure. This redirection of the flow of *prana* has a calming effect on the mind, strengthens our inner focus, and also directs our awareness toward higher consciousness. As such, using the *bandhas* can be likened to the temporary damming of a river for it to be redirected more usefully.

The three major *bandhas* to be used in conjunction with certain yoga *asana* and *pranayama* are as follows.

Mula Bandha – Root Lock

The Sanskrit words *mula* and *bandha* mean "root" and "lock" so *Mula Bandha* refers to the energetic "lock" near *muladhara chakra*, at the base of the spine. Also called the "perineum lock", this involves gently contracting the muscles of the pelvic floor, which lifts and tones the organs of the pelvis. Think of the squeezing action that you would take to stop urinating mid-stream and you have a good idea of the feeling you are trying to achieve. There is no external sign when you are applying this *bandha* so no photograph can illustrate it.

Uddiyana Bandha – Abdominal Lock

The Sanskrit term *uddiyana* means to "fly upward"
– an appropriate notion for this lock which,
when applied by contracting the upper abdominal
muscles, causes the diaphragm to "fly upward", or
rise, toward the chest. It helps to direct *prana* into the
sushumna nadi (the central energy pathway in the spine) so
that it flows upward to *sahasrara chakra*, thus helping you on
your journey toward self-realization. To apply this lock, think of
gently sucking your stomach in and up as much as possible.

CAUTION: Practise only on an empty stomach. Pregnant women
and those suffering from high blood pressure, heart problems
and stomach ulcers should avoid it.

Jalandhara Bandha – Throat Lock

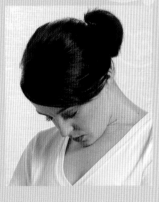

This lock is achieved by lowering and
pressing the chin to the sternum, while
the chest is raised with the inhaling breath
toward the chin. The Sanskrit terms *jalan*
and *dhara* mean "net" and "stream" so this
lock seals off the network of *nadis* in the
neck, preventing the "stream" of *prana*
between the *chakras*, and instead directing
it into the *sushumna nadi*. This promotes an
increased sense of calm.

CAUTION: Those with high blood pressure, heart problems, mental stress
and migraine should only practise this under the guidance of an experienced
yoga teacher.

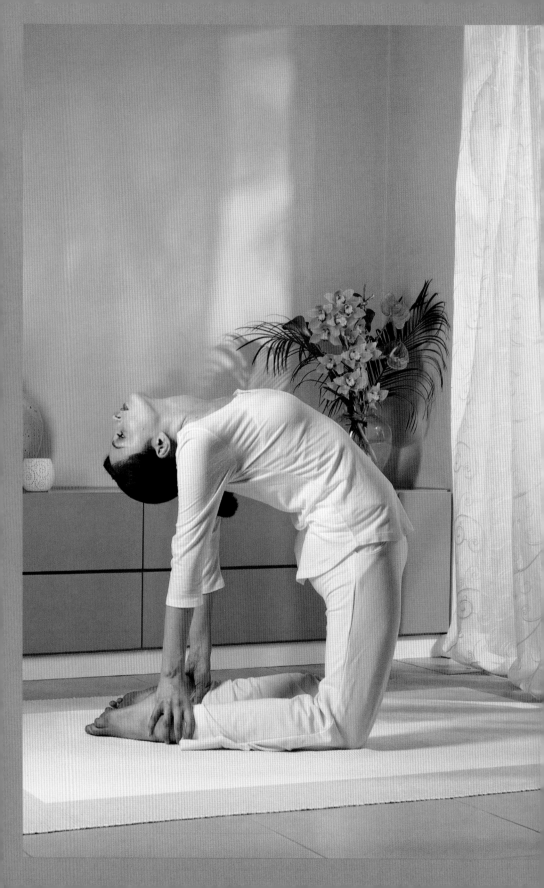

CHAPTER 4

ASANA PRACTICE

POSTURES TO REVITALIZE YOUR BODY'S ENERGY

Regularly doing the yoga postures (*asanas*) in this chapter will not only help to enhance your physical health. The sequences are also designed to awaken the subtle energy in your body — so that it can be consciously directed from the spine to the higher brain centres in the meditation practices to follow, encouraging you to find your sense of inner peace and stillness.

Firstly, you will be led through warm-up exercises, which limber up the body. Next, you will be guided through the Sun Salutation Sequence (*Surya Namaskara*), which invigorates and balances all the body's systems. Next, there are two sequences to choose between: an Energizing Morning Sequence and a Relaxing Evening Sequence. Finally, there is a Cool-Down Sequence, which can be added to the end of either a morning or evening practice. Ideally, this whole set of sequences would be completed before doing any of the rest of the practices in the book. However, if you don't have time for this, simply choose the most suitable sequence for the time, whether the Sun Salutation to reinvigorate you, the Morning Sequence to set you up for the day, the Evening Sequence to wind down or the Cool-Down Sequence to really switch off and relax.

WARMING UP

Before beginning your yoga routine proper, practise at least a few of the warm-up exercises that follow to limber the spine, loosen your muscles and prepare your mind. Make sure you do each movement slowly, with concentration, coordinating your breathing (both in and out through the nose) with your movements. There is instruction given with each exercise as to when you should inhale or exhale.

❀

Benefits of the warm-up

It is good to get into the habit of giving yourself time to warm up before starting your Yoga Meditation routine proper, as doing the exercises on the pages that follow will confer the following benefits:

• Standing Body Stretch stretches the spine and relaxes the whole body.

• Crossing Arms Above Head relaxes the shoulders, stretches the chest muscles and encourages deep breathing.

• Upper Body Side Bend stretches and strengthens the muscles along the sides of the abdomen and back.

• Upper Body Twist promotes flexibility of the spine, and relaxes both the upper and lower back muscles.

• Chair Pose strengthens the leg muscles and stretches the arms.

• Upper Body Swing invigorates the entire body, deepening breathing and promoting flexibility in the back and hips.

Preparing the body

❀

1 Standing Body Stretch

Stand with your legs together and your arms at your side. Inhaling, rise up onto your toes and stretch your arms above your head, so that you stretch your whole body. Exhaling, slowly lower your heels and return to the starting position. Repeat five times in total.

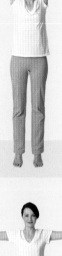

2 Crossing Arms Above Head

a) Stand with your legs slightly wider than hip-width apart, your arms relaxed by your sides and your back straight. Inhaling, raise your arms straight out to shoulder level at each side, palms facing downward.

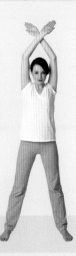

b) Exhaling, cross your arms above your head, palms facing forward. Inhaling, lower your arms to your sides and return to the starting position. Repeat Steps a and b ten times in total.

3 Upper Body Side Bend

Standing with your legs slightly wider than hip-width apart, clasp your fingers behind your head and push your elbows slightly back. Exhaling, bend your upper body sideways to the left, ensuring that you don't lean either backward or forward. Inhaling, return to the centre. Exhaling, bend your upper body sideways to the right, again ensuring that you don't lean either backward or forward. Inhaling, return to the centre. Repeat three times on each side in total.

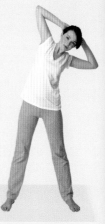

4 Upper Body Twist

Standing with your legs slightly wider than hip-width apart, clasp your fingers behind your head and push your elbows slightly back. Inhale deeply, then as you exhale, turn your upper body to the left. Inhale and turn back to the centre. Exhale, turn to the right; then inhale, return to the centre. Repeat three times.

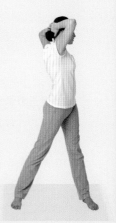

5 Chair pose

Standing with your feet hip-width apart, hold your arms straight out in front of you at shoulder level and inhale. Exhaling, slowly lower your body by bending your knees into a squat position, as if you are about to sit on a chair. Keep your feet flat on the floor, with your knees over your ankles. Hold for a count of five breaths, then inhale and return to the standing position. Repeat five times.

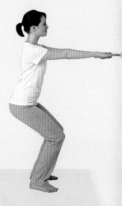

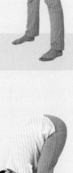

6   Upper Body Swing

a) Stand with your feet wide apart. Inhaling deeply, raise both arms straight above your head. Allow your hands to relax and drop forward.

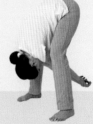

b) Then, exhaling deeply through your mouth, stretch your arms and upper body forward, swinging them as far as is comfortable between your legs, taking care not to lock your knees. Inhaling, swing slowly back up to standing upright, with your hands above your head. Repeat this swinging movement ten times in total.

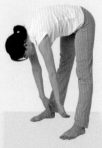

c) Then, breathing normally, allow your body to relax and hang forward for three breaths before slowly raising your body upright on an inhalation, with your arms stretched above your head. Finally, exhale and lower your arms slowly to bring them to your sides.

CAUTION: Do not practise this exercise if you suffer from high blood pressure or have a slipped disc or other back issues.

SUN SALUTATION SEQUENCE

The flowing yoga sequence known as the Sun Salutation (*Surya Namaskara* in Sanskrit) is an invaluable series of postures that can be done at any time, whether as a complete exercise in its own right, or as part of a wider routine as advised in this book, because it:

- greatly enhances flexibility in the spine and limbs
- stretches and strengthens all the major muscle groups in the body
- stimulates circulation
- helps to overcome fatigue
- encourages the healthy flow of *prana* throughout the body
- helps to coordinate the body, mind and breath, bringing focus to your mind in preparation for meditation.

The sequence can be done either slowly, in a meditative way, or at a faster pace to really energize the body. The important thing is to practise with awareness and concentration, and to try to synchronize your breathing (both in and out through the nose, or *Ujjayi* breathing, see pages 98–9) with the physical movements. If this seems difficult at first, focus on the body positions initially and then, once these are familiar, begin to coordinate your movements with your breath.

To add another dimension, more experienced practitioners might like to concentrate on the *chakra* that corresponds to each position. These are listed in the steps that follow, and information on the *chakras* can be found on pages 34–41.

CAUTION: Avoid the sequence on pages 69–71 if you suffer from high blood pressure, dizziness, slipped disc or other back issues.

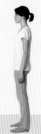

1 Mountain Pose – *Tadasana*

Begin by standing tall with your feet together and your arms relaxed by your sides. Close your eyes and become aware of the natural rhythm of your breath – in through your nose and out through your nose. CONCENTRATION: *muladhara* (root) *chakra*.

2 Prayer Pose – *Pranamasana*

Exhaling, join your palms together in the classical prayer position in front of your heart. Feel this movement begin to "centre" your energy. CONCENTRATION: *anahata* (heart) *chakra*.

3 Upward Salute – *Urdhva Hastasana*

Open your eyes. Inhaling, slowly sweep your arms out to the sides and overhead, keeping your arms straight and ending up with your palms pressed together or facing each other. Lift your chest and arch your back slightly. CONCENTRATION: *vishuddhi* (throat) *chakra*.

4 Standing Forward Bend: *Uttanasana*

Exhaling, slowly fold into a standing forward bend, aiming to place your hands either side of your feet in line with your toes. If your legs feel tight, bend your knees slightly. Lengthen your spine as you release your head, shoulders and arms toward the floor. CONCENTRATION: *svadhisthana* (sacral) *chakra*.

5 Rider's Lunge – *Ashwa Sanchalasana*

Inhaling, bend both knees and lower your right knee to the ground as you stretch the leg back. At the same time keep your left foot between your hands, and your knee directly over your ankle. Raise your head and look up. CONCENTRATION: *ajna* (third eye) *chakra*.

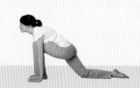

6 Plank – *Phalakasana*

Holding your breath, extend your left leg back so that it is aligned with your right leg. Keep both legs straight and allow your arms to support your upper body, while your toes and feet support your lower body. Lengthen from the base of your spine through to the top of your head, extending your heels back.

CONCENTRATION: *manipura* (solar plexus) *chakra.*

7 Salute with Eight Points – *Ashtanga Namaskara*

Exhaling, bend and lower first your knees to the floor, then your chest and chin too, ensuring that your shoulders and fingertips align as you bend your arms and that your elbows don't go out to the sides. Your buttocks should remain raised.

CONCENTRATION: *manipura* (solar plexus) *chakra.*

8 Cobra – *Bhujangasana*

Keeping your slightly bent elbows close to your body and your shoulders relaxed, push your hands gently into the floor to raise your head and upper body, arching your spine backward, while keeping your hips, legs and the tops of your feet on the floor. Direct your gaze between your eyebrows.

CONCENTRATION: *svadhisthana* (sacral) *chakra.*

9 Downward Dog – *Adho-Mukha-Svanasana*

Exhaling, tuck your toes under, raise your hips to the sky, straighten your arms and push your body backward. Allow your head to relax between your arms and press your heels toward the floor.

CONCENTRATION: *vishuddhi* (throat) *chakra.*

10 Rider's Lunge – *Ashwa Sanchalasana*

Inhaling, lunge your right leg forward, bringing your right foot between your hands. Lower your left knee to the floor and stretch your left leg back, resting the top of your foot flat on the floor. Look up. CONCENTRATION: *ajna* (third eye) *chakra*.

11 Standing Forward Bend – *Uttanasana*

Exhaling, step your left leg forward to meet the right and fold your body forward from the hip joints, bringing your forehead toward your shins. Bend your legs slightly, if you need to, for comfort. CONCENTRATION: *svadhisthana* (sacral) *chakra*.

12 Upward Salute – *Urdhva Hastasana*

Inhaling, slowly raise your upper body, first with your arms outstretched in front of you and then overhead, with the palms pressed together or facing each other. Slightly arch your spine backward. CONCENTRATION: *vishuddhi* (throat) *chakra*.

13 Mountain Pose – *Tadasana*

Exhaling, lower your arms to your sides and and look straight ahead. Take one or two slow deep breaths here to centre yourself. CONCENTRATION: *anahata* (heart) *chakra*.

Next repeat the entire sequence, this time on the opposite side: taking your left knee to the floor in Step 5 and your right knee to the floor in Step 10. This completes one "round" of the Sun Salutation. It is good to begin with six complete rounds and gradually progress to 12 rounds.

ENERGIZING MORNING SEQUENCE

The sequence of yoga postures that follows will really stretch your spine and legs, awakening your body and filling it with vitality for the day ahead. Be sure to practise slowly, with awareness, and try to tune into the energy running through your spine as you relax into each pose. Breathe deeply and smoothly in and out through your nose unless stated otherwise.

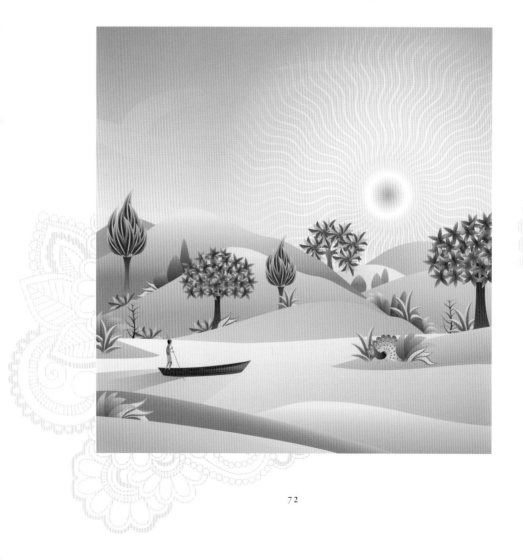

1   Mountain Pose – *Tadasana*

Stand tall with your feet together and your arms by your sides, relax your eyes and face, and look straight ahead.

2   Standing Forward Bend – *Uttanasana*

Exhaling, bend forward from your hips, taking your upper body toward your legs. If you are unable to place your hands on your feet (as shown), try holding your opposite elbows with your hands and pulling them down to lengthen your trunk. Hold for five breaths. Then, inhaling, come up slowly.

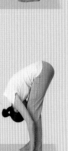

3   Triangle Pose – *Trikonasana*

Stand with your feet over 1m (about 4ft) apart and parallel. Extend your arms out to the sides at shoulder height. Turn your left foot out by 90 degrees and your right foot in by about 15 degrees. Exhaling, bend your body down to the left, aiming to hold your ankle or as low down your leg as you can. Stretch your right arm up and turn the palm to face forward. Keeping your right hip rolled back, turn your head to look up at your hand. Hold for five breaths. Then inhaling, come up slowly. Turn your feet to the front, then repeat on the other side, this time with your right foot turned out and your left foot in.

4 Side-Angle Pose – *Parsvakonasana*

Stand with your feet over 1m (about 4ft) apart and parallel again. Turn your left foot 90 degrees out and your right foot slightly in. Exhaling, bend your left leg to a right angle and lower your body to the left, placing your left forearm on your left thigh. Stretch your right arm overhead, palm facing forward, turn your head to look up at your arm, and feel the stretch down the right side of your body. Hold for five breaths. Then inhaling, come up. Turn your feet to the front, then repeat on the other side.

5 Warrior – *Virabhadrasana*

Stand with your feet over 1m (about 4ft) apart and parallel again. Turn your left foot out 90 degrees and your right foot in 45 degrees, then turn your hips to face the same direction as your left toes. Exhaling, bring your arms overhead, palms together, stretch upward and look up at your hands. Hold for five breaths. Then, inhaling, come up. Turn your feet to the front, then repeat on the other side.

6 Sideways Intense Stretch – *Parsvottanasana*

Stand with your feet just less than 1m (about 3ft) apart. Turn your left foot out 90 degrees and your right foot in 45 degrees, then turn your hips to face the same direction as your left toes. Inhaling, stretch your body up, then, exhaling, bend forward from your hips, over the left leg, reaching your hands toward the floor (or as low on your leg as they reach). Hold for five breaths. Then, inhaling, slowly come up. Turn your feet to the front, then repeat on the other side.

7   Camel Pose – *Ustrasana*

Kneel on the floor with your legs hip-width apart and your body in a vertical line from your knees upward. Tuck your tailbone under and draw your abdomen in. Place your hands on your hips, with your elbows back, to lift your chest. Inhaling, lengthen your spine and circle your right arm up and behind to touch the right heel. Repeat with your left arm so that your spine ends up arched backward, keeping your abs tight and your thighs vertical. If you are unable to reach your heels (or it is causing discomfort), place your hands on your hips and gently arch back. Hold for five breaths. Then, inhaling, slowly come up and sit on your heels.

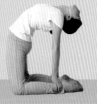

8   Seated Forward Bend – *Paschimottanasana*

Sit on the floor with your legs together, stretched out in front of you and your spine upright. Press your thighs down and extend through your heels. Exhaling, bend forward from your hips and clasp your feet, ankles or shins, depending on your flexibility. Aim to rest your upper body and head on your legs. Hold for five breaths.
Then, inhaling, slowly come up to sitting.

"The secret of health for both mind and body is not to mourn for the past, worry about the future, or anticipate troubles, but to live in the present moment wisely and earnestly."

Paramhansa Yogananda

Relaxing Evening Sequence

The sequence of yoga postures that follows will help you to unwind from your daily activities by freeing tensions from your body, awakening energy in your spine and increasing the blood circulation to your brain to both vitalize and relax you for meditation. Breathe deeply and smoothly in and out through your nose, unless otherwise stated.

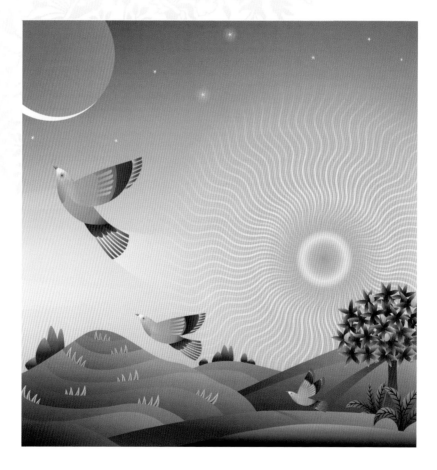

1 Upward Thunderbolt Pose – *Urdhva Vajrasana*

a) Kneel on the floor, with your buttocks on your heels, your hands on your thighs and your body upright but relaxed.

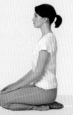

b) Inhaling, raise both your arms above your head, stretching your spine slightly back, and expanding your chest to open your heart and lungs. Look toward your hands, hold for five breaths, then release.

2 Hare Pose – *Shashankasana*

Exhaling, bend your body forward, reaching your arms in front of you and resting your forehead on the floor. Keep your buttocks on your heels if you can. Hold for five breaths, then release.

3 Cobra Pose – *Bhujangasana*

Lie down on your stomach, resting the tops of your feet on the floor. Inhaling, press your hips into the floor and raise your upper body, supporting yourself with your hands under your shoulders, elbows tucked in. Arch your back slightly and look up, pressing your shoulders down and back. Hold for five breaths, then release.

4 Downward Dog – *Adho-Mukha-Svanasana*

Exhaling, tuck your toes under, straighten your arms and legs, and raise your hips high. Push your heels into the floor and your buttocks into the air. Relax your head between your arms and direct your gaze toward your knees. Hold for five breaths, then release.

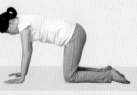

5 Cat Pose – *Majariasana*

a) Come down onto all fours, aligning your knees directly under your hips and your hands directly under your shoulders, with your back in a relaxed straight line.

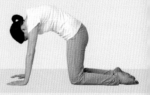

b) Inhaling deeply, arch down your lower spine and extend your head, neck and chest upward. Push down through the hands to lift your upper spine and look directly ahead.

c) Exhaling, tuck your tailbone under, draw your abdomen in, bow your head to look toward your navel and arch up your whole spine.

d) Repeat the arching down (Step b) and arching up (Step c) movement five times in total.

6 Child's Pose – *Balasana*

Inhale as you sit back on your heels. Exhale as you fold your upper body forward to rest your forehead on the floor if you can. Rest your arms by your sides, palms facing upward. Take your attention inward and focus your awareness on your breath. Rest here for ten breaths, then very slowly sit up into Thunderbolt Pose (see page 54).

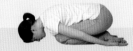

7 Corpse Pose – *Shavasana*

If you are finishing your practice here, lie down on your back with your head, neck and spine in a nice straight line, your feet a comfortable distance apart and your arms slightly away from the sides of your body, palms facing up. Let your feet fall loosely to the sides and remain completely still. Close your eyes and relax your whole body. Maintain the inner focus of your mind by being aware of the natural rhythm of your breathing. Remain here for as long as you feel the need. If, however, you have time to continue to the Cool Down Sequence, you can skip this posture here as you will do it at the end of your cool down.

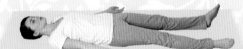

COOL DOWN SEQUENCE

The following soothing sequence of mainly inverted yoga postures (where the head is lower than the heart) will benefit the whole body, massaging and nourishing your internal organs by increasing the blood supply to them. It will also enhance physical and mental relaxation in preparation for meditation. Breathe deeply and smoothly in and out through your nose unless stated otherwise.

❁

Benefits of inverted poses

While inverted poses in yoga are often seen as difficult, the benefits of gently mastering these poses are manifold. Reversing the action of gravity on the body has a number of useful health-promoting outcomes.

As mentioned above, inverted poses invigorate the entire body and provide support for internal organs. However, these poses also deepen breathing, relax the nervous system, and promote flexibility in the back and hips. The Shoulderstand can help with headaches too, as the muscles in the neck and shoulders are released and benefit from a greater supply of blood.

CAUTION: Do not practise the inverted poses on the pages that follow (Steps 2 to 5 – Shoulderstand to Bridge) during menstruation, pregnancy or if suffering from high blood pressure, a neck injury or eye problems such as a detached retina or glaucoma. Fish Pose is fine to practise during menstruation but is not suitable during pregnancy.

1   Lying Down, Legs Out Straight

Lie on your back with your legs straight out, your arms by your sides and your palms on the floor. Tuck your chin in. Breathe rhythmically from your abdomen.

2   Shoulderstand – *Sarvangasana*

Inhaling, raise your legs to 90 degrees, keeping them straight. Press your hands into the floor to raise your hips and legs, and bring your hands onto your lower back for support, fingers pointing inward and thumbs around the hips. Continue to raise your legs and hips higher, moving your hands closer to your shoulder blades to support the balance. Aim to have your body in a vertical line, elbows tucked in, bring your chin close to your chest, and relax your feet. Hold for up to three minutes, breathing rhythmically from your abdomen. If this is too challenging, you can do Half Shoulderstand (*Ardha Sarvangasana*) instead: just extend your legs over your head at a comfortable angle, resting your hips in your hands and keeping the weight of your body on your upper back, not your neck.

3   Plough Pose – *Halasana*

Exhaling, slowly lower both legs over your head, aiming to rest your toes on the floor but keeping your hips lifted and pressing your arms into the floor behind your back, palms down. Hold for up to three minutes, breathing rhythmically from your abdomen. If this is too challenging, try placing two folded blankets under your shoulders, bend your legs behind you and place your feet onto a support, such as a small, sturdy stool of an appropriate height.

4 Knee-to-ear Pose – *Karnapidasana*

Exhaling, lower your knees either side of your ears if you can and place your arms behind your knees and your hands over your ears. Hold for one minute, breathing slowly. To come out of the pose, extend your arms on the floor behind your back, press your palms flat into the floor and lower your spine, vertebra by vertebra. Then slowly lower your legs so that you're lying on your back, with your legs together and arms by your sides, palms on the floor. If this is too challenging, simply move straight from Plough (Step 3) to Bridge (Step 5).

5 Bridge – *Setubandhasana*

a) Still lying on your back, with your arms by your sides, bend your knees up, placing your feet flat on the floor, about 50cm (20in) apart and parallel. Be careful not to let your knees fall inwards.

b) Exhaling, place your hands on your lower back, fingers turned inward and thumbs on your sides, keeping your elbows on the floor. Push your hips and thighs upward, arch your spine and do not let your knees push forward over your toes. Press both feet evenly into the floor. Hold the pose for five breaths. Then, breathing slowly, exhale and release.

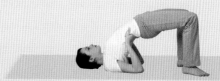

6   Fish Pose – *Matsyasana*

Lying on your back with your legs together, arms by your sides and palms on the floor, slide your arms under your body so that your hands, palms down, are beneath your buttocks. Inhaling, raise yourself up onto your elbows and lift your chest as high as you can. Gently extend your head back and lower the top of your head toward the floor. Hold the pose for about half the time you held the Shoulderstand (as a counterpose). To come out of the pose, keep the weight on your elbows, inhale, raise your head and lower your spine gradually to the floor.

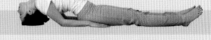

7   Corpse Pose – *Shavasana*

Lie on your back with your head, neck and spine in a nice straight line. Place your feet about 60cm (2ft) apart, relaxing them out to the sides. Your arms should be at 45 degrees to your body, palms facing up. Inhale, then tense all the muscles in your body and hold the breath for a few seconds, before exhaling, completely letting go of all tension. Close your eyes and focus your awareness on your breathing: as you inhale the abdomen rises, as you exhale the abdomen falls. Relax for as long as you can afford, feeling the energy flowing throughout your body. You will now be in a much more ready state for meditation.

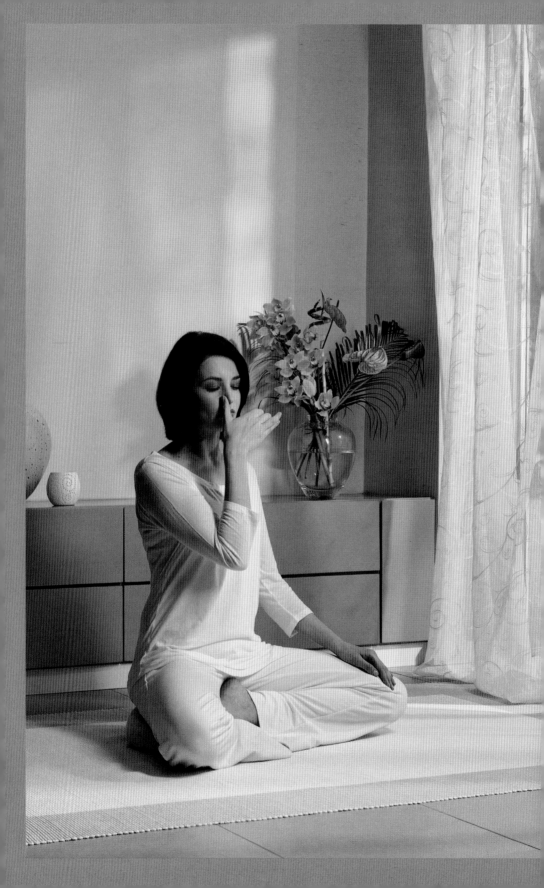

CHAPTER 5

PURIFICATION PRACTICE

TECHNIQUES TO CLEANSE YOUR BODY AND MIND

Both a healthy body and a healthy mind are required to sustain the increased levels of energy needed for Yoga Meditation. It is therefore important that any impurities – whether physical (known as *malas*) or mental (known as *vikshepas*), such as doubt, inattention, laziness and pleasure-seeking – are removed before meditation.

When the purification practices in this chapter – *Nadi Shodhana* (Alternate Nostril Breathing), *Agnisara Kriya* (Activating the Digestive Fire), *Kapalabhati* (Skull-shining Breath) and *Ashvini Mudra* (Horse Gesture) – are regularly performed, preferably daily, they will purify the body's energy channels, strengthen the digestion, burn up toxins, massage the internal organs, awaken the life energies of the body, and cleanse and calm the mind in preparation for meditation.

Aim to do the four purifications as part of your regular yoga practice (preferably in the morning) – after your yoga postures and before your *pranayama* and meditation. Doing this regularly for at least three to six months will allow you to experience the optimum benefits of increased energy and clarity of mind.

NADI SHODHANA: ALTERNATE NOSTRIL BREATHING

This important exercise – also commonly known as *Anuloma Viloma* – purifies all the energy channels of both the physical and astral bodies so that *prana* can flow smoothly; *nadi* is Sanskrit for "flow", and *shodhana* for "purification". The exercise also balances breathing between the left and right nostrils and activity between the left and right brain hemispheres, which has a calming effect on the nervous system. When the flow of air becomes equal in the nostrils, the flow of energy in the *ida* and *pingala nadis* is also equalized, which allows *prana* to flow in the central *sushumna nadi*, centring the mind for the purpose of meditation.

Regular practice will increase your capacity for focused concentration and meditation. It is best to start using a ratio of 4:8:8 – inhaling for a count of four, holding the breath for eight, exhaling for eight.

❀

Vishnu Mudra

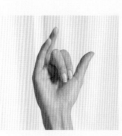

This *mudra*, which involves folding your middle and index fingers into your palm and keeping your thumb and ring and little fingers extended, is used in *Nadi Shodhana* to help to contain *prana* within the body. The right hand is usually used to perform this *mudra*.

Practising Nadi Shodhana

❀

1 Sit in a comfortable meditation pose (see pages 52–7), close your eyes and relax your whole body.

2 Relax your left hand on your left knee, palm upward.

3 Raise your right hand and position it in *Vishnu Mudra* (see below left).

4 Exhale and close your right nostril with your thumb.

5 Inhale slowly and smoothly through the left nostril for a count of four.

6 Gently close your left nostril with your ring and little fingers so that both nostrils are now closed, and hold your breath for a count of eight.

7 Release your thumb and exhale slowly through your right nostril for a count of eight.

8 Remain with the left nostril closed and inhale through your right nostril to a count of four.

9 Close both nostrils and hold your breath to a count of eight.

10 Release your left nostril and exhale through it for a count of eight. This completes one full round; repeat from Step 5 to start the next round. Practise five to ten rounds in total daily. Over a period of time, gradually aim to increase to 25 rounds. Once you've progressed to 25 rounds at this 4:8:8 ratio, revert to five to ten rounds, but this time trying a 5:10:10 ratio.

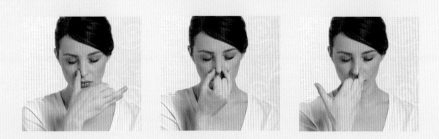

AGNISARA KRIYA: ACTIVATING THE DIGESTIVE FIRE

Agni is Sanskrit for "fire", *sara* means "essence" and *kriya* means "action". This purification practice is therefore a means of stimulating the "essence of fire", which is thought to be at the navel in yogic terms; this creates internal heat to rekindle the digestive fire. It is also an effective exercise for toning the abdominal muscles. Spiritually, it activates *manipura chakra* at the navel, which frees us from negative energies and imbues us with vitality.

Only ever do the exercises on pages 89–90 on an empty stomach, and after evacuation of the bowels. If you are new to the practice, it is best to do just Stage 1 first, then gradually progress to the more advanced Stages 2 and 3 as your abdominal muscles become stronger. Stages 2 and 3 are, however, best learned under the guidance of an experienced yoga teacher.

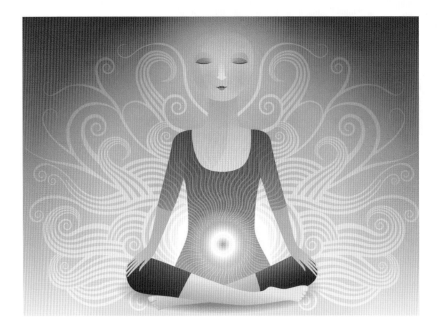

Practising Agnisara Kriya

❀

Stage 1: Abdominal Squeeze

1 Stand with your feet slightly wider than hip-width apart. Bend your knees and lean forward, pressing your hands on your thighs just above your knees, and keeping your arms straight.

2 Inhale deeply. Then relax your abdomen, and as you exhale deeply, firmly contract your abdominal muscles, pressing the navel toward the spine. Comfortably hold the abdominal contraction with your breath held out for a few seconds. As you inhale, relax and allow the abdomen to return to its normal position. Repeat five to ten times.

Stage 2: Abdominal Pumping

1 Remain leaning forward, with your hands pressed on your thighs just above your knees, arms straight.

2 Inhale deeply, then, exhaling deeply and slowly, contract the lower abdominal muscles just above your pubic bone, pulling them firmly inward and upward. This also creates a strong upward pressure in the perineum area between the genitals and anus. Continue exhaling, while contracting the abdominal wall up toward the ribcage. As you complete the exhalation, inhale and, without pause, in a wave-like motion, slowly release the contraction from the upper to the lower abdomen.

3 On your next exhalation, once again contract first your lower, then your upper abdominal muscles. Then, holding your breath for as long as you comfortably can without strain, pump your abdominal muscles in and out in quick succession. At first, aim to do about 20 "pumps". Then inhale, relax and stand upright again. As you become more experienced, you can gradually increase to doing ten rounds of 20 pumps, taking a short break between each round.

Stage 3: Abdominal Rolling (*Lauliki Nauli*)

1 Bend your knees again and lean forward, pressing your hands on your thighs just above your knees, and keeping your arms straight.

2 Exhale deeply, and firmly contract your abdominal muscles, bringing the navel toward the spine. This is *Uddiyana Bandha* (see page 61).

3 Maintaining this lock, press your hands into your legs and give a forward and slightly downward thrust to the abdominal portion between the navel and the pubic bone. This helps to contract the rectus abdominus muscles – the two long vertical rows of muscle running down the centre of the abdomen – keeping the other muscles of the abdomen in a relaxed condition. Equal hand pressure on your legs further helps you to achieve the isolation of the rectus abdominus muscles.

4 Once you can achieve this initial isolation of these muscles, try to isolate just the right rectus muscle (*Dakshina Nauli*) by leaning your body forward, tilting your torso slightly to the right and putting extra pressure on the right hand.

5 Then try to isolate the left rectus muscle (*Vama Nauli*) by leaning slightly to the left while increasing pressure on the left hand.

6 Finally, start trying to move each one from side to side so they move or "roll" in a wave-like movement in quick succession. Begin by doing five rolls to the right and five to the left.

CAUTION: Do not practise any of these exercises during menstruation (*Agnisara Kriya* stimulates the upward flow of pranic energy, which is counter to the natural downward cleansing flow), while pregnant or after an abdominal operation, or if you have a stomach disease, cardiovascular disease or high blood pressure.

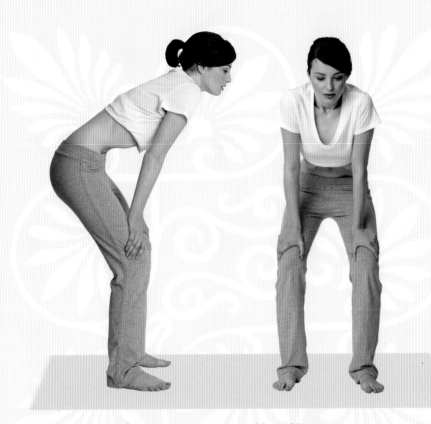

This shows Stage 2 of Agnisara Kriya practice — Abdominal Pumping — in action.

The art of Abdominal Rolling

❀

It will take time and perseverance to master Abdominal Rolling as it is an advanced exercise that requires voluntary control of the central abdominal muscles. You will need to learn how to isolate, contract and rotate the rectus muscles in a churning motion while maintaining a static posture. This practice is therefore best learned under the expertise of an adept yoga teacher. However, it is included here because, once learned, it is a valuable practice that contributes toward the awakening of dormant *kundalini*, helping it to ascend through the *sushumna* to the crown *chakra*.

KAPALABHATI:
SKULL-SHINING BREATH

Kapala is Sanskrit for "skull" and *bhati* means "shine". The practice of *Kapalabhati*, which involves a series of rapid, active exhalations and passive, effortless inhalations, therefore literally "shines" or purifies the cavities within the skull, invigorating the brain with a massaging effect, rejuvenating the nervous system, and awakening dormant centres responsible for subtle perception. It expels more carbon dioxide and other waste gases from the cells and lungs than normal breathing. If you feel dizzy at any point while doing it, simply stop, sit quietly and breathe normally. When you feel ready to begin again, breathe with awareness and less forcibly.

1 Sit in a comfortable meditation pose (see pages 52–7), palms on your knees, close your eyes, relax your whole body and breathe deeply, in and out through your nose.

2 Begin actively emphasizing your exhalation by contracting your abdomen, so that you feel your diaphragm lift, pushing the air out of your lungs forcefully through both nostrils. This will create a vacuum so that the passive inhalation happens naturally. This is one respiration.

3 Continue by rapidly exhaling and inhaling through both nostrils without pausing, making each exhalation short, strong and powerful and each inhalation light, relaxed and effortless. Aim to keep the muscles of your face relaxed.

4 Start with three rounds of ten to 20 rapid respirations. Aim to add ten respirations per "round" each week until you reach 120 respirations per round.

CAUTION: Those suffering from heart problems, high blood pressure, epilepsy, nausea or fainting should not practise *Kapalabhati*.

ASHVINI MUDRA: HORSE GESTURE

The traditional practice of *Ashvini Mudra*, meaning "horse gesture", is named after a subtle internal dilation and contraction of the anal sphincter muscles that a horse is known to make several times once it has evacuated its bowels. Repeatedly contracting the anal sphincter muscles in this way acts as a perineal seal, conserving *prana* and redirecting it to the higher *chakras*, preparing the mind for meditation. The exercise also promotes overall strength and vigour and is a good preparatory practice for *Mula Bandha*, the root or anal lock (see page 60). It also has physical benefits of strengthening the anal muscles and helps in counteracting disorders such as constipation, piles and prolapsed uterus or rectum.

1 Kneel in Thunderbolt Pose (see page 54) with your head, neck and spine upright and aligned. Rest your palms on your thighs.

2 Inhale deeply, hold your breath and contract your gluteal muscles, pelvic diaphragm and anal sphincter for a few seconds, then release. The feeling is like the squeezing of your back passage to stop yourself going to the loo. Repeat the contraction and release rapidly as many times as you can hold your breath comfortably without strain.

3 Repeat Step 2 twice more so that you do three rounds of contractions in total. Aim to slowly and gradually work your way up to being able to do 30 contractions in one go, then 60, being careful not to strain in any way.

NOTE: To make it easier to get the feeling when you first do it, you might want to try it lying down on your back with your legs and feet together. Any posture that pulls the hips together will make it easier.

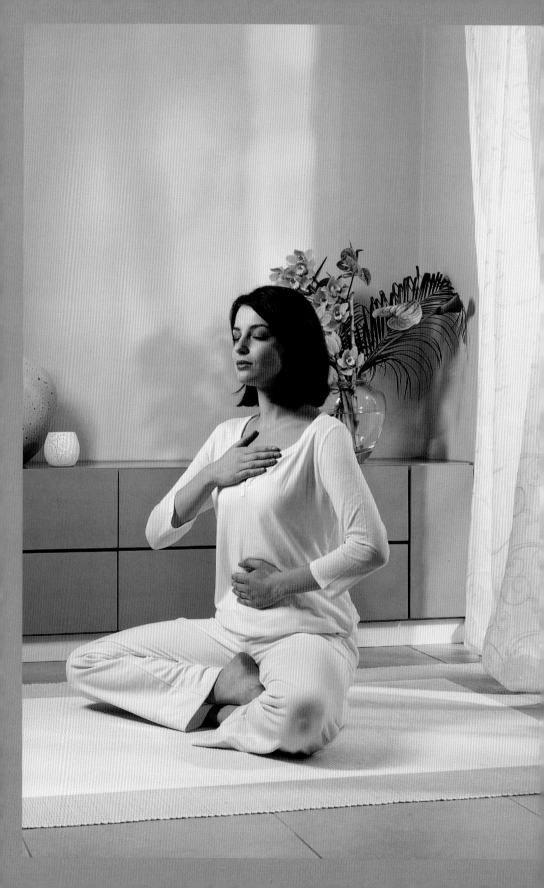

CHAPTER 6

PRANAYAMA PRACTICE

REGULATING YOUR VITAL LIFE-ENERGY THROUGH BREATH

The techniques in this chapter aim to get you more attuned to the vital energy within your body via the powerful vehicle of the breath, which is the most tangible sign of internal pranic activity.

After all, the Sanskrit word *pranayama* – one of the Eight Limbs of Yoga – is composed of two parts: *prana*, meaning the vital energy within us, and *ayama*, meaning to regulate or extend. *Pranayama* practices therefore act as a means to regulate and harmonize the movement of the vital energy in your body. As any movement of thought in the mind is believed to arise from the movement of *prana*, gaining the ability to regulate and still the *prana* will allow you to still and focus your mind, too – helping to avoid "monkey mind" symptoms, where thoughts jump all over the place.

In the majority of types of *pranayama* breathing, just as in normal breathing, it is standard to breathe both in and out through the nose, unless otherwise instructed.

Pranayama is best practised in the early morning – after the purification practices (see pages 84–93) and before meditation (see pages 106–137). However, many of the practices that follow can be done any time to help access a feeling of increased calm and peace.

The Complete Yogic Breath

The Complete Yogic Breath is a fundamental *pranayama* practice that will help to restore deeper, balanced breathing, leading to enhanced physical and mental relaxation and making you feel more centred within. It will also help to relieve fatigue, refreshing the whole body by increasing oxygen intake. As it involves breathing in a smooth, uninterrupted transition from the abdomen, to the mid-chest, to the upper chest, it also teaches you how to maximize your lung capacity so that you use the entire respiratory system. The Complete Yogic Breath is especially useful in times of stress for helping to calm the nervous system and to replenish energy levels.

Practising the Complete Yogic Breath

❦

Stage 1: Inhalation

1 Sit in your choice of comfortable meditation pose (see pages 52–7). Close your eyes and relax the body.

2 Abdomen: Exhale deeply through the nose, contracting the abdomen to squeeze out all the air from the lungs. Then inhale slowly through the nose, keeping the lower part of the abdomen contracted while expanding the abdomen above the navel slightly.

3 Mid-chest: At the end of the upper-abdomen expansion, allow the breath to come into your mid-chest to expand that area.

4 Upper chest: Continue drawing the breath into the higher lobes of the lungs, so that it lifts and expands your upper chest, causing your collarbones and shoulders to rise. Your lungs should now be completely filled with air.

Stage 2: Breath Retention

1 Hold the breath in for a few seconds, gently tilting the head forward onto the upper chest in *Jalandhara Bandha* (Throat Lock; see page 61). Only hold *Jalandhara Bandha* for as long as is comfortable while you are holding your breath.

Stage 3: Exhalation

1 Release *Jalandhara Bandha* by raising your head.

2 Upper chest: Start to exhale through your nose, relaxing your upper chest, so that your collarbones and shoulders lower naturally back into their normal position.

3 Mid-chest: Continue exhaling so that you feel your mid-chest relax.

4 Abdomen: Continue exhaling until you feel the release of your abdomen so that your lower ribs begin to soften inward. You can place one hand on your abdomen and the other on your upper chest, in order to feel the breath as it leaves first your chest and then your abdomen.

This completes one Complete Yogic Breath. Repeat for a total of five to ten full breaths, then return to normal breathing.

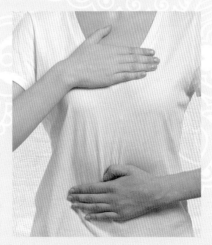

NOTE: The Complete Yogic Breath can be practised at any time, and can also be done in a standing position or lying down on your back.

Ujjayi pranayama: Victorious Breath

Ujjayi breathing has two distinct qualities: the soft sibilant sound it produces and its smooth, even flow. In deep sleep this type of breathing occurs naturally. The technique slows the breath down so is conducive to calming the mind and improving concentration for deep meditation. It can be practised as an exercise in its own right when you need to relax or as part of a series of Yoga Meditation practices.

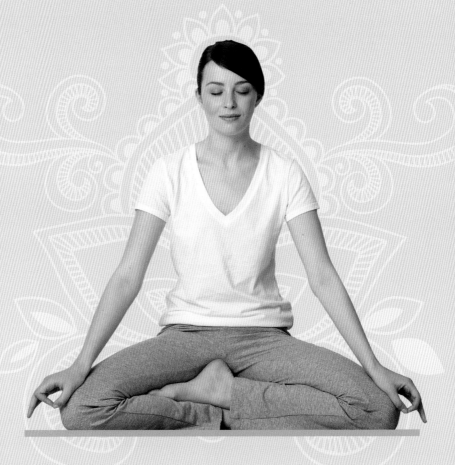

Practising Ujjayi

❀

1 Sit in your choice of comfortable meditation pose (see pages 52–7). Close your eyes, relax your body and take a few deep breaths. Inhale deeply through your nose and tense your whole body, then exhale through your mouth and let go of all tension. Place your hands, palms down, on your knees in *Jnana Mudra* (see page 59).

2 Close your mouth and inhale through both nostrils smoothly and evenly, with the glottis partially closed, so that the breath makes a "haaa" sound within the throat; the glottis is the opening between the vocal cords, at the upper part of the windpipe. This is similar to the feeling you experience when you yawn (see also box below). During the inhalation keep the abdominal muscles slightly contracted and expand the lungs with air, until the chest protudes forward like that of a victorious warrior.

3 Now exhale slowly with a smooth, deep and continuous breath through both nostrils, listening to the subtle sibilant "haaa" sound that the outgoing breath makes. The abdominal muscles should naturally be more contracted than during inhalation. Make the exhalation last twice as long as the inhalation. This is one round of *Ujjayi* breathing.

4 Do five rounds and increase by two rounds each week until you reach 20.

❀

Mastering the art of Ujjayi

To understand the feeling of the *Ujjayi* breath better, try exhaling through your mouth and whispering a long "haaa" sound, feeling how the breath creates a soothing sensation along the back of your windpipe. Now close your mouth while making this sound and slowly inhale with the same feeling in your throat, then breathe out through your nose with the same steady internal "haaa" sound.

BHASTRIKA PRANAYAMA: BELLOWS BREATH

This invigorating breathing technique – known as "Bellows Breath", as the body's diaphragm is made to pump like the bellows that a blacksmith uses to fan air into a fire – has both a purifying and energizing effect on the body. It not only cleanses the *nadis* but also helps in the activation of *manipura chakra* and optimizing the flow of *kundalini*, in preparation for meditation. It oxygenates and purifies the bloodstream and brings you back into balance with your body. It also enhances optimum functioning of the glands.

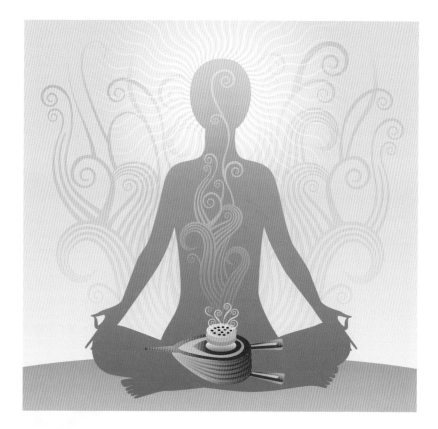

Practising Bhastrika Pranayama

❀

1 Sit in your choice of comfortable meditation pose (see pages 52–7). Close your eyes and relax your body.

2 Place your right hand in *Vishnu Mudra* (see page 86), by folding your index and middle fingers in toward your palm, and close your right nostril with your right thumb.

3 Inhale and exhale quite forcefully ten times through the left nostril, so that the expulsions of breath follow one another in rapid succession. This will cause the abdomen to move in and out in a pull-and-push action.

4 Next, take a long, deep inhalation and exhalation through the left nostril.

5 Now close your left nostril with your fingers, release your thumb from your right nostril, and inhale and exhale ten times rapidly.

6 Then take a long, deep inhalation and exhalation through your right nostril.

7 Release *Vishnu Mudra* and return your hand to your knee.

8 Continue the bellows breath by rapidly breathing in and out through both nostrils for ten breaths.

9 Close your left nostril again with your index and little fingers, inhale deeply through the right nostril and hold the breath in for as long as is comfortable without strain, tilting your chin toward your chest to apply *Jalandhara Bandha* (see page 61) and also applying *Mula Bandha* (see page 60). Place your awareness at *muladhara chakra* (see page 38) at the base of the spine, where your *kundalini* lies.

10 Slowly release *Jalandhara Bandha*, then *Mula Bandha*, and exhale slowly and smoothly through your left nostril. Release *Vishnu Mudra*.

Bhramari Pranayama: Bee-breathing Technique

During the exhalation stage of this breathing exercise, a buzzing sound is made like a bee; the Sanskrit term *bhramari* means "large bee". Regularly doing this practice, using this soothing sound, will quickly help to calm your thoughts and nerves, and promote concentration, preparing you for deep meditation in order to bring you into contact with your true sense of self and thereby promote a deep sense of inner peace.

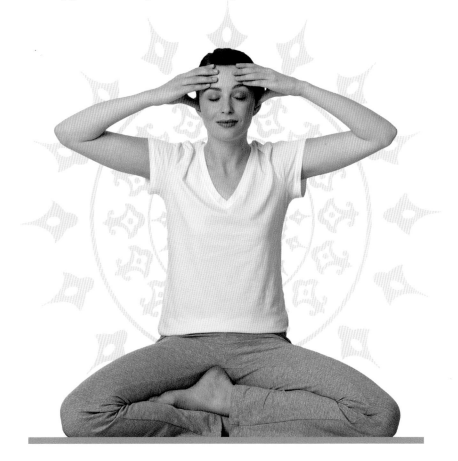

Practising Bhramari Pranayama

❅

1   Sit in your choice of comfortable meditation pose (see pages 52–7). Close your eyes, relax your body and rest your hands on your knees in either *Jnana Mudra* or *Chin Mudra* (see pages 58–9).

2   Inhale deeply through your nose, using *Ujjayi* breath (see pages 98–9), creating a mild suction effect in the throat and feeling a cool sensation there. Visualize drawing this cool current of energy up from the base of your spine to the top of your spine.

3   Hold the breath in, apply *Jalandhara Bandha* (see page 61), bring your focused attention to your spiritual eye, the mid-point between your eyebrows, and close your ears with your thumbs by pressing the ear-flaps, while resting the fingers of each hand on your forehead.

4   After about five seconds, simultaneously release *Jalandhara Bandha*, remove your hands from your forehead (while keeping your ears closed), and slowly exhale through your nose, with your mouth closed, but with your teeth slightly separated. As you exhale, make a long, deep, even humming sound, like that of a bee. Feel the sound vibrating throughout your brain, while concentrating on *sahasrara chakra* at the top of your head. The longer the humming exhalation, the more relaxed you are likely to feel but do not force the breath beyond its natural capacity.

5   This completes one round of *Bhramari Pranayama*. Sit still with the ears still closed, breathe normally and focus on the inner sound, which arises from the heart region. Aim to practise five rounds at first, taking one or two normal breaths between each round. Over time, you can aim to increase to ten rounds.

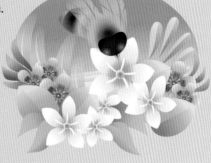

KUNDALINI PRANAYAMA:
NADI SHODHANA AND OM MANTRA

Regularly doing this *pranayama* practice, which uses the *Nadi Shodhana* technique (see pages 86–7) in a 3:12:6 ratio along with the *Om* mantra (see pages 130–33), helps to awaken the energy in the spine. The resonating vibration of *Om* attunes us with our true nature and higher reality.

If it feels uncomfortable to hold your breath for the 12 *Oms* in Step 4 (see right), it's best not to practise this exercise just yet. Instead, spend more time practising *Nadi Shodhana*, which will gradually build up your stamina.

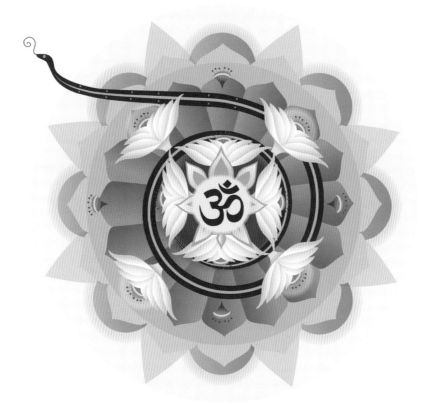

Practising Kundalini Pranayama

❀

1   Sit in your choice of comfortable meditation pose (see pages 52–7), close
your eyes and relax your whole body, taking a few deep breaths. Inhale
deeply and tense your whole body, then exhale and let go of all tension
and relax. Place your hands, palms down, on your knees, with the index
fingers and thumbs lightly touching in the *Chin Mudra* (see page 58).

2   Close your eyes and direct your inner gaze to the spiritual eye in the
middle of your forehead (see page 40). Relax here with your awareness on
the breath for a few minutes, then bring your awareness to *muladhara
chakra* (see page 38) at the base of your spine.

3   Raise your right hand and fold your middle and index fingers into your
palm, keeping your thumb, ring and little fingers extended in the *Vishnu
Mudra* for practising *Nadi Shodhana* (see page 86). Close the right nostril
with your right thumb, exhale, and then inhale through the left nostril
for a mental count of three *Oms*. As you inhale, visualize drawing in *prana*.

4   Gently close your left nostril with your ring and little finger so that both
nostrils are now closed and hold your breath for a mental count of 12
Oms. As you retain the breath, feel that you are sending the current of
pranic energy down through your spine into *muladhara chakra*, at the
base of your spine.

5   Release your thumb and exhale slowly through the right nostril for a
mental count of six *Oms*. As you exhale, feel a sense of calm within.

6   Now, remaining with the left nostril closed, start to repeat the process
in reverse: inhale for three *Oms* through your right nostril, close both
nostrils and hold your breath for 12 *Oms*, and release your left nostril to
exhale through it for six *Oms*. This completes one full round.

7   Practise five complete rounds (Steps 3–6) with concentration. After
finishing, remain sitting quietly with your awareness at your spiritual eye
for as long as you are able to.

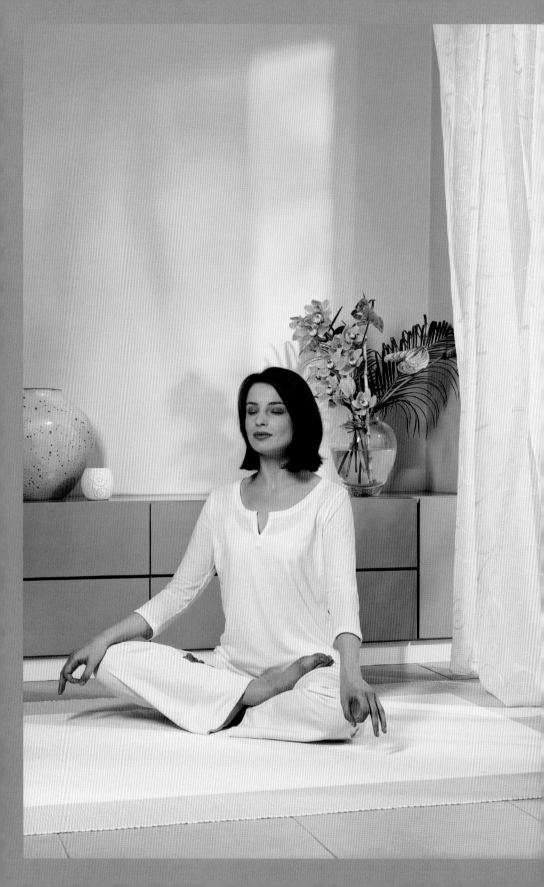

ॐ

CHAPTER 7

MEDITATION PRACTICE

EXPERIENCING THE BLISS OF YOUR TRUE DIVINE NATURE

As discussed throughout this book, meditation is the ideal tool to enhance a sense of calm, fulfilment and well-being in your life, and the only way to come to know your true divine nature, which is *Sat-Chit-Ananda* — ever-existing, ever-conscious, ever-new bliss.

The meditation practices within this chapter have been hand-picked from the Kriya Yoga tradition (see page 12) to help you to move toward these valuable goals.

Firstly, we will explore the key ways of focusing the mind for meditation. Then we will present a range of exercises that will help you to focus your concentration, awaken energy within your spine, tune in to your *chakras* to promote enhanced flow of *prana*, and engage with your natural breath in recognition of the fact that you are, in essence, at one with the universe. Finally, we will present the art and practice of Ultimate Bliss Yoga Meditation — the key practice to which all the other exercises in this book have been leading.

If you can do as many of these meditation practices as often as possible — at least three times a week — you will soon be experiencing a deep joy in life that is entirely independent of the external world.

FOCUSING THE MIND

Focusing the mind for effective meditation means not allowing it to become restless or scattered in all directions, and instead holding it to one point of focus. Concentration itself is a narrowing of the field of attention, making the mind one-pointed.

In our current, fast-paced technological age, things often tend to be orientated toward outward action and constant seeking rather than inner reflection. As such, the world keeps our mind and senses continuously active and preoccupied, and we can easily lose any sense of our true identity or our spiritual goal in life.

Meditation is like a bird. It needs two equally strong wings to fly: constant awareness of the spiritual goal of life on one side – realizing that our true inner nature is divine – and a focused mind on the other side. Until you have trained your mind to be free from its habit of continually moving outward, you will make little progress in meditation.

Here follows a grounding in a range of the most effective tools for focusing the mind in order to enhance your Yoga Meditation practice, as well as your quality of life in general. The main techniques are:

- Breathing – in yoga, the breath is the most commonly used tool for focusing the mind. Consider what happens when you concentrate intensely to hear a whisper; your breath stops. This illustrates that our mind and breath are inseparable.
- Visualization – in visualization, sense, object and mind are brought together to form an internal image on which the mind can focus.
- Mantras and chanting – mantras are sacred sounds that have powerful effects on us by focusing our mental energy; chanting mantras draws the mind inward to a focused concentration.
- Steady gazing – concentration on an object such as a candle flame, an *Om* symbol or a picture of a spiritual master focuses the mind inward.

❀

Opening the heart

Love is the highest state and final goal of spiritual realization. It therefore makes sense that you have to open your heart as well as focus your mind during Yoga Meditation. Without love and devotion, your meditation practice would be mechanical, dry and of little worth. Practising meditation with love and devotion can lead the mind beyond mere intellectual knowledge to an experience of the blissful self, which constitutes true wisdom. For love is the divine within you. Love is your inner source and potential. Love is your true nature.

So how can you cultivate love? Think of a garden: to grow flowers, first you need to create a space. And so it is with love; first you need to clear the tangled weeds of desire, attachment, anger, greed and fear from your heart. The soil of your heart must then be watered and fertilized by cultivating compassion, care and understanding for all. Next, when the tender shoots of service and devotion sprout up, you must keep them free from the insects of selfish egoism.

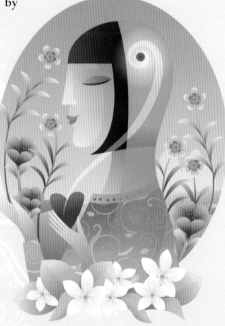

Just as you can see the moon only by reflected rays of light from the sun, similarly, you can see the divine only through rays of love. By opening your heart and cultivating divine love within you, the dark clouds disperse. Then you will recognize that the same divinity resides in others as in yourself.

BREATHING

A highly effective way to keep your mind in the present moment is to give it the mental object of watching the breath, which is constantly flowing in and out through your nostrils.

You can concentrate on the breath by focusing your attention on the rising and falling of your abdomen, or the expansion and contraction of the ribcage, as you inhale and exhale. The Complete Yogic Breath (see pages 96–7) can help with awareness of this movement.

Alternatively, it can be useful to focus on the sensation of the breath at the point where it enters your nostrils. This is, for example, the basis of the *Hong Sau* technique (see pages 122–5). In this meditation, you go on to watch the naturally occurring spaces between the breaths, in which the mind becomes very still. By uniting your mind with the breath in this way, the mind will start to stay focused in the present moment.

There are many other ways of working with the breath, such as counting a certain number of breaths in and out, and visualizing it going to certain parts of your body, but all breath techniques work on the same premise of giving the mind a specific object on which to focus.

VISUALIZATION

Visualization is a powerful tool for helping to focus your mind for meditation, whether bringing to mind a calm scene, a visual representation of your *prana* or *chakras*, a spiritual guide or any other positive image, as it transports your mind to one particular scene and allows it to sit there, with positive intention.

It is important to be as relaxed as possible when you use visualization. Create the relevant pictures in your mind as vividly as you can. Pay attention to every detail. The more lifelike the visualization, the better the results you will get. But remember that people receive images in different ways. For example, you may receive your impressions through physical sensations, emotions or thoughts rather than pictures. So do not dismiss your impression just because you cannot "see" the images. Your visualization is valid, whatever form the experience may take. For example, sensing the warmth of the sun on your skin, or feeling healing light infusing the cells of your body can be just as useful as visualizing colour and light. Examples within the meditation practices on the following pages that involve visualization are *Tratak* (see page 113), where you picture a candle flame in your mind in Step 3; and *Jyoti Mudra* (see pages 128–9), where you are asked to see the inner light of the spiritual eye.

❀

Simple visualization to calm and focus your mind

You can use this simple visualization any time that your thoughts feel scattered and you want to come back into the present moment. Sitting relaxed in a calm, quiet place, begin by taking a few deep breaths to bring your mind to the present moment. Visualize yourself walking barefoot on a beach. It is early evening and the white sand is still warm from the day's sun. Above, the sky is fading to deep blue. As the sun begins to set, the horizon is streaked with shades of orange, red and purple. Listen to the waves roll in from the sea and break onto the white sand, sparkling and foaming about your feet. Feel the warm, wet sand between your toes. Smell the salt water. Feel the soft breeze from the sea on your skin. Listen to the far-off cry of a seagull. To your left is a large rock. Slowly walk to it, sit down on it and close your eyes. You feel a great sense of peace and tranquillity in the present moment, a feeling of being connected to all life. Enjoy and stay immersed in this inner peace for as long as you can.

MANTRAS AND CHANTING

Reciting a mantra is one of the most powerful ways of focusing the mind. Deriving from the Sanskrit for "that which protects or liberates the mind", a mantra is a unique and sacred sound (letter, syllable, word or phrase) that has a radiant energy, which can transform the mind.

Just as a white cloth takes on the colour of the dye in which it is soaked, so does the mind absorb the qualities of the sacred sound vibration of the mantra that is recited. Whether said silently inside your head, whispered or chanted out loud, mantras help to internalize the mind and have the ability to transform the consciousness of the reciter.

The practice of reciting a mantra is called *japa* (repetition). When you practise correctly, with attentive awareness, *japa* will gradually calm and integrate your mind, so that your awareness vibrates with the mantra. This naturally leads you into a deeper state of stillness in meditation, where you go beyond the mind to rest in your true divine nature.

When mantras are chanted aloud, the rhythmical vibrations produced by continually repeating them regulate the unsteady vibrations of the five sheaths (see pages 30–33). It is best if such chanting begins aloud, then gradually softens, until it fades into silent, internal chanting.

The source of all sound vibrations, and probably the most well known mantra, is the sacred Primordial Creative Vibration and Divine Power, known as *Om* or *Aum* (see page 117). The sincere repetition of *Om* produces thought waves that correspond to those of the supreme reality. Using the seed mantras related to each of the seven *chakras* (see pages 118–19) enhances concentration and energy levels. The *Hum* (pronounced "hoom") mantra (see pages 120–21) enhances and protects the power of all other mantras, as well as having a fiery energy that destroys negativity. And the *Hong Sau* mantra (see pages 122–5) calms the mind and helps to awaken the energy in your *chakras*. Whatever the mantra used, it will help the mind to turn inward and therefore become much more calm.

STEADY GAZING

The following concentration exercise, known as *Tratak*, can be done any time. It steadies the wandering mind and enhances willpower. The Sanskrit word *Tratak* means "to gaze continuously at an object without blinking". Here we suggest gazing at a flame, but you could use any other object with positive associations.

1   Sit in a comfortable meditation posture in a darkened room, with a lighted candle about an arm's length in front of you, at about chest height.

2   Fix both your gaze and mental focus at the mid-point of the flame where it is brightest for as long as possible without blinking, until your eyes begin to become tired. At the start, practise only for about one minute, then increase to a few minutes over a period of time.

3   End by closing your eyes and visualizing the flame internally in the space between your eyebrows for one minute. Then, repeat the whole process two more times. When you have finished your practice, rub your palms together until they are warm. Place them over your eyes to relax and soothe them. Then, when you feel ready, lower your hands.

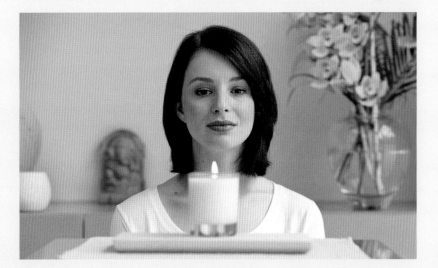

MAHA MUDRA:
AWAKENING ENERGY IN YOUR SPINE

When practised properly, the powerful Hatha Yoga technique of *Maha Mudra* (meaning "great gesture" in Sanskrit) provides not only a range of physical benefits, such as stimulating digestion and easing constipation, but also balances and opens the *ida* and *pingala nadis* (see pages 44–5), encouraging the life-force to flow upward in the central *nadi*, the *sushumna*.

When the right big toe is grasped in Stage 1 of *Maha Mudra* (see right), *pingala nadi* is opened and activated. And when the left big toe is grasped in Stage 2 (see page 116), *ida nadi* is opened and activated. When both toes are pulled simultaneously in Stage 3, the spine becomes magnetized with *prana* flowing into the *sushumna*, which will bring deeper awareness and concentration to your meditation.

NOTE: The version of *Maha Mudra* presented on pages 115–117 includes a knee position slightly modified from the traditional Hatha Yoga version in that it does not require a rotation. If you have any problems with your knee, you may therefore find this posture easier to practise.

❀

Benefits of bandhas

The two bandhas – *Mula Bandha* and *Jalandhara Bandha* (see pages 60–61) – that are held as part of *Maha Mudra* retain energy in the spine, so that the energy can be directed upward into the higher centres in the brain leading to an increased sense of vitality and balance.

Stage 1

❀

1   Sit upright with your head, neck and spine aligned and your legs stretched out in front of you. Bend your left leg with the knee pointing forward and sit on your left foot, with the heel pressing against the perineum (between the genitals and anus) forming an anal lock (*Mula Bandha*; see page 60). Breathe in *Ujjayi* breath (see pages 98–9) if you are familiar with it, or breathe normally if not.

2   Bend your right leg and place the foot flat on the floor. Then, interlocking the fingers of both hands together, stretch forward, clasp your hands around your right knee and draw the thigh in against your torso, or as close as possible. Keep your spine straight in this position, inhale slowly to a count of ten to 15 and feel that you are drawing a cool current of *prana* up your spine.

3   Then, holding the breath, stretch your right leg out in front of you, bend forward, and with interlocked hands, grasp your big toe and gently pull, so that you extend your trunk forward and your forehead toward the knee. If this is uncomfortable, bend the knee slightly. The important thing is to feel the spine stretching and a sensation of energy rising through it. As you do so, bring your chin toward your neck to apply the throat lock (*Jalandhara Bandha*; see page 61), and with your attention at your spiritual eye, or *ajna chakra*, between your eyes (see page 40), mentally chant *Om* six to 12 times. Feel a sensation of energy rising up through the spine and pulsating at your spiritual eye, radiating waves of bliss through the brain.

4 Release the throat lock, move your clasped hands to just below your right knee and draw your knee back up against your torso, while slowly exhaling to a count of ten to 15. With your awareness in your spine, feel that you are drawing a warm current of energy down through it.

Stage 2

❀

Now change sides and repeat Stage 1, starting by tucking your right foot under and pulling your left knee to the torso with your clasped hands.

Stage 3

❀

1 Sit upright with your knees bent and clasp your hands (fingers interlocked) around your knees, pulling your thighs against your torso. Inhale for a slow count of ten to 15, feeling that you are drawing a cool current of *prana* up the spine.

2 Now, holding your breath, stretch both legs out together in front of you, grasp your big toes with your interlocked hands and pull on them, stretching your torso forward and feeling the stretch in your spine. Apply the throat lock again and bring your forehead toward your knees. Meanwhile, focus your attention at your spiritual eye,

between the eyebrows, and mentally chant *Om* six to 12 times. You may feel a sensation of energy rising up through the spine followed by pulsating at the spiritual eye, resulting in waves of bliss radiating throughout the brain.

3   Release the throat lock and slowly exhale to a count of ten to 15. Keeping your awareness in the spine, see if you feel a warm current of pranic energy flowing down the spine. Then bring your knees and thighs back up against your torso, by pulling on the knees with clasped hands. Relax and return to normal breathing.

These three stages complete one round of *Maha Mudra*. Practise three complete rounds. As you progress with this practice, you may increase the number of rounds to 12.

❁

Significance and pronunciation of Om

The primal vibratory sound *Om* (see also pages 130–33) helps to awaken energy in the spine and stimulate the brain cells when chanted. When the word is sounded it is *Om*. In this exercise, the correct pronunciation of *Om* is like a long, drawn-out version of "home" without pronouncing the "h". Give equal measure to both the "o" and "m" sounds, and close with the sound "mmm". However, it is also occasionally written as *Aum*. The three separate letter sounds in this variant represent the three states of consciousness, as well as the divine trinity of Brahma, Vishnu and Shiva.

CHANTING THE BIJA MANTRAS:
AWAKENING THE CHAKRAS

As explored on page 112, chanting is an effective way to enhance energy throughout the body, as well as to focus the mind. The meditation practice opposite activates the *chakras* using the sound vibration of the particular mantras associated with each one. These are known as *bija* or seed mantras. Each "seed" mantra clears its *chakra* of any blockages so that it can function efficiently, allowing you to reach a deeper meditative state. Below are the seed mantras and musical notes (if you choose to sing them) for the first six *chakras*. The seventh *chakra*, *sahasrara* (crown) *chakra* is not included as the other six need to be cleared first in order to access the ineffable experience of the seventh *chakra*. It is important to pronounce all the mantras in the list containing an "a" with a long "aaa" sound.

	CHAKRA	LOCATION	SEED MANTRA	MUSICAL NOTE
	AJNA	forehead	Om	F
	VISHUDDHI	throat	Ham	E flat
	ANAHATA	heart	Yam	D
	MANIPURA	navel	Ram	B flat
	SVADHISTHANA	genital area	Vam	A
	MULADHARA	base of spine	Lam	G

Practising the bija mantras

❀

1 Sit in your choice of comfortable meditation posture (see page 52–7) with your head, neck and spine aligned. Close your eyes.

2 Bring your awareness to your *muladhara chakra,* located at the base of the spine. Inhale deeply and as you exhale, repeatedly chant aloud the *bija* mantra "Lam". Feel the mantra vibrating at the *chakra* as you chant "Lam, Lam, Lam" for as long as your exhalation lasts.

3 Next, bring your awareness to the second *chakra*, *svadhisthana*, located at the genital area. Inhale deeply and as you exhale, chant the *bija* mantra "Vam". Feel the mantra vibrating at the *svadhisthana chakra.*

4 Slowly work your way through the other *chakras* on the chart opposite, chanting the corresponding seed mantra and feeling the vibration at the relevant *chakra* centre each time you do so.

5 Once you have completed your chanting, focusing on the *ajna chakra*, start working your way through the list in reverse order, chanting each seed mantra again while focusing on the related *chakra* area. Start with "Om" for a second time at the ajna chakra, and finish with "Lam" at *muladhara chakra.*

❀

Mentally chanting the bija mantra

The exercise above can also be done by chanting each seed mantra internally instead of out loud. Inwardly chanting the mantras through the *chakras* places more emphasis on the calming, meditative effect of the practice, while chanting them aloud puts more emphasis on its vibrant, energizing aspect.

CHANTING THE HUM MANTRA: INCREASING PRANA

It is said that the Hindu god Lord Shiva used the *Hum* mantra (pronounced "hoom") to project fire from his third eye in order to burn desires and negativity. This mantra therefore brings a fire energy and power to all who chant it by helping to increase *prana* in the body and to activate the potent life-force known as *kundalini*. This helps to combat any negative feelings, as well as easing fatigue and lethargy.

In the exercise that follows, the *Hum* mantra is chanted after a *chakra's* seed mantra, in order to enhance its energy. Then, by adding *Om* at the start of a seed mantra, you can make it even more effective for opening the mind for deep meditation. The exercise opposite can either be done after the *bija* mantra exercise (see page 119) or as a technique in its own right.

	CHAKRA	LOCATION	MANTRA	MUSICAL NOTE
	AJNA	forehead	Om Ksham Hum	F
	VISHUDDHI	throat	Om Ham Hum	E flat
	ANAHATA	heart	Om Yam Hum	D
	MANIPURA	navel	Om Ram Hum	B flat
	SVADHISTHANA	genital area	Om Vam Hum	A
	MULADHARA	base of spine	Om Lam Hum	G

Practising the Hum mantra

❀

1   Sit in your choice of comfortable meditation posture (see pages 52–7) with your eyes closed and focus your awareness at the point between your eyebrows, known as your spiritual eye.

2   Transfer your awareness to *muladhara chakra*, at the base of your spine, and chant aloud the mantra "Om Lam Hum" six to nine times, feeling it resonating at the site of this *chakra*. Sit quietly and continue to feel the vibration of the mantra even when you stop the actual chanting.

3   Next, transfer your awareness to your *svadhisthana chakra* at the genital area, and chant aloud the mantra "Om Vam Hum" six to nine times, feeling it resonating there. Again, sit quietly and sense the vibration of the mantra once when you stop the actual chanting.

4   Slowly work your way through the other *chakras* shown opposite, chanting the corresponding mantra each time, and feeling the vibration at the location of the *chakra*. Be sure to pause for a short silence between each mantra.

NOTE: Lam, Vam, Ram, Yam, Ham and Ksham should be sounded with a long "aaa" sound. *Om* should be sounded as "ong". *Hum* should be sounded as "hoom".

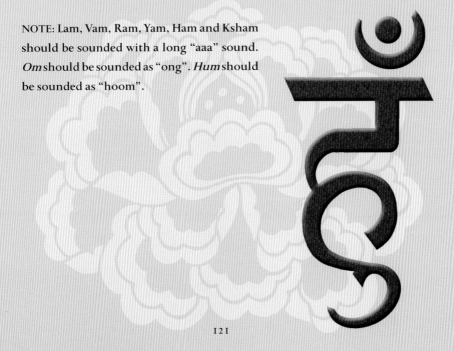

HONG SAU MEDITATION:
I AM HE, THE ABSOLUTE

Hong Sau (pronounced "Hong Saw") is an ancient Sanskrit mantra for calming the mind and deepening concentration. Repetition of this mantra stills restless thoughts, withdraws the mind from the senses and calms *prana* in the body. *Hong Sau* means "I am He" or "I, the manifest self, am He, the Absolute." By internally repeating *Hong Sau* in harmony with your breathing during meditation – *hong* on the inhalation and *sau* on the exhalation – you affirm that the individual self is one with the Infinite Spirit.

Hong Sau is considered to be the natural, subtle sound of the breath:

- *Hong* vibrates with the inhalation, representing the contraction of consciousness and corresponds to the ascending current in the *ida nadi* (see pages 44–5)
- *Sau* vibrates with the exhalation, representing the expansion of consciousness into pure unity and corresponds to the descending current in the *pingala nadi*.

Over the course of 24 hours, the breath is said to flow in and out 21,600 times in a continuous mantra of *Hong Sau*. In yoga, such continuous subconscious recitation is called *ajapa-japa*, while *japa* is the term used to describe the conscious mental recitation in the technique that follows.

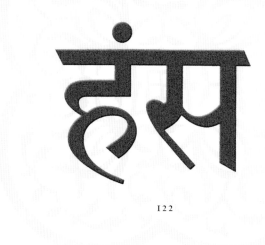

Hong Sau preparation

❁

As well as forming a useful calming sequence in its own right, the steps below will prepare both your body and your mind for the *Hong Sau* technique on the next page.

1   Sit in your choice of comfortable meditation posture (see pages 52–7) with your head, neck and spine aligned. Inhale deeply, hold the breath and tense all the muscles in your body. Hold both the breath and the tension in your muscles for a few seconds, then simultaneously release them and relax. Repeat the process of tensing and relaxing three times.

2   Continue to remain relaxed as you practise what is called *Loma Pranayama*: a three-part equal-breath-ratio exercise, breathing through both nostrils. Inhale for a count of 12, hold your breath for a count of 12, exhale for a count of 12 (12:12:12). If this is not within your lung capacity, halve the counts to six. Do this nine times at first and gradually increase over a period of time to anything up to 27 rounds.

3   Now concentrate your relaxed attention at the point between your eyebrows (your spiritual eye, or ajna chakra; see page 40). Let go of all thoughts and be totally centred in the present moment. Place your hands, palms upward, on your knees in Chin Mudra (see page 58), close your eyes and place your focus on your natural breath, as you inhale and exhale, inhale and exhale … If your mind wanders, gently bring it back to the practice of watching your breath with awareness.

Hong Sau technique

❀

1 Now with your body and mind still, and your eyes closed, gently lift your gaze upward to the point between the eyebrows, and look calmly into your spiritual eye, or *ajna chakra* – the seat of your intuition and of omnipresent perception.

2 Feel the natural breath flow in and out of your nostrils and try to establish the point where it feels strongest. Once you have found this point (usually just inside the tip of the nose), observe the breath that passes it with precision, one split second after another. In this way, continuous awareness will eventually result.

3 Then begin to feel the sensation of the air higher in the nostrils, up by the point between your eyebrows, and focus on this area. As your concentration deepens, your breathing will begin to slow down, and you will be able to focus on it more clearly, with fewer interruptions.

4 Inhale deeply, then slowly exhale. As the next inhalation naturally flows into your nostrils, feel the breath where it enters, and with your inner focus, mentally follow the breath with the mantra *Hong*. Imagine that the breath itself is making this sound.

5 As your breath flows out naturally, mentally follow it with the mantra *Sau* (pronounced "saw"). Once again, feel that your subtle breathing is silently making the sound of its own accord.

6 Continuing to focus on your spiritual eye, between your eyebrows, mentally follow each inhalation with the mantra *Hong*, and each exhalation with the mantra *Sau*. When the mind is united with the flow of the breath, you will be able to truly experience the present moment.

7 As you go deeper into this practice, you may notice that there is a natural space or pause, a point of complete stillness, between each inhalation and exhalation. This is the space of the innermost Self. Softly focus your awareness on these pauses. As your mind becomes more calm, notice the spaces extending and enjoy the experience of expansion while inwardly

gazing into your spiritual eye. Then, when the breath naturally returns, continue with the practice of *Hong Sau* for as long as it feels natural, or in the beginning up to 15 minutes.

8 Once you finish, try to maintain a sense of that inner space from your meditation for as long as possible, allowing the calmness to permeate your everyday consciousness.

NOTE: It is important to make no attempt to control the breath during the *Hong Sau* technique. This is not a yoga breathing exercise. It is simply a matter of being consciously aware of the breath, with your concentration on the *Hong Sau* mantra.

❀

The spiritual eye of intuitive perception

In deep meditation it is possible to naturally see and experience the gold-, blue-, and white-coloured light of the spiritual eye, or *ajna chakra*. But while you are working toward this, you might want to try *visualizing* it in order to add another dimension to your meditation:

- An outer gold ring of light represents cosmic energy.
- A sphere of blue light represents the omnipresent intelligence of the divine in creation.
- A central silver-white star represents infinite spirit or cosmic consciousness, a doorway to the infinite.

NAVI KRIYA: AWAKENING PRANA IN THE NAVEL CENTRE

Navi Kriya (pronounced as "Nabi Kriya") is one of the original Kriya Yoga techniques, taught by Lahiri Mahasaya, who learned the supreme science of Kriya Yoga meditation from Mahavatar Babaji, the great Himalayan yogi (see page 12).

The purpose of this Yoga Meditation technique is to stimulate and awaken the *prana* at *manipura chakra*, in the navel centre, and draw the energy from here up the spine to the spiritual eye, or *ajna chakra*, elevating your consciousness above the lower *chakras* to access a more meditative state. It is essential to be established in *ajna chakra* before you can be liberated in *sahasrara*, the crown *chakra* at the top of the head.

Practising Navi Kriya

❀

1 Sit in your choice of comfortable meditation position (see pages 52–7) with your head, neck and spine aligned. Relax your whole body, close your eyes and bring your attention for a moment to the point between the eyebrows, at your spiritual eye, or *ajna chakra*.

2 Then bring your awareness to *muladhara chakra*, at the base of your spine, and slowly inhale and mentally chant *Om* as if you were sending the mantra's energy into this *chakra*.

3 Repeat this internal chanting of the mantra *Om* at each of your ascending *chakras* in succession, sending the energy there each time:
   • *svadhisthana* – at the genital area
   • *manipura* – at your navel
   • *anahata* – at your heart
   • *vishuddhi* – at your throat
   • the medulla oblongata – the negative pole of *ajna chakra* (see page 40),

which is located at the back of your head, below the base or rear of the brain
• the spiritual eye *chakra* (positive pole of *ajna chakra*), which is located
between your eyebrows.

4 Slowly tilt your chin down towards your neck, forming a throat lock (see
page 61), and bring your awareness to *manipura* chakra at your navel.

5 As you continue to breathe normally, mentally chant *Om* 100 times to
activate this *chakra* and bring energy up from the lower two chakras:
muladhara and *svadhisthana*. A calm energy is usually perceived
gathering around the navel; this is the *prana* current called *samana vayu*
guiding your *prana* into the subtle *sushumna* channel (see page 44).

6 Maintaining your awareness at *manipura chakra*, and with your inner
gaze at the point between your eyebrows, release the throat lock, raise
your chin to the upright position, and slowly tilt your head back as far as
is comfortable without strain. See if you can feel your energy moving into
the area at the base of your skull known as the medulla oblongata, and
then back down through your spine to *manipura chakra* at your navel
centre.

7 Holding your head back in this tilted position, mentally chant *Om* 25
times, directing the mantra's energy into the counterpoint of the navel
on the back of your spine.

8 Now slowly raise your head to its normal position, and with concentration,
once again mentally chant *Om* successively at each of the six *chakras*, this
time starting at the *ajna chakra* and moving downward: *ajna, vishuddhi,
anahata, manipura, svadhisthana* and *muladhara chakras*.

8 This completes one round of *Navi Kriya*. Aim to practise six to 12 rounds,
then sit quietly for a few moments with your inward attention at your
spiritual eye. When you return to your normal activities, carry this
natural sense of inner stillness and energy with you to give you the inner
strength to overcome life's trials and tribulations.

Jyoti Mudra:
Awakening the Inner Light

Jyoti Mudra — meaning "gesture of light" — is a technique by which you can enhance your sense of inner peace and wisdom by focusing on the inner light that radiates from the spiritual eye, or *ajna chakra* (see also page 40). In Yogic texts this *mudra* is commonly referred to as *Yoni Mudra*, the Sanskrit word *yoni* denoting the womb of creation because, like the baby in the womb, anyone practising *Yoni Mudra* becomes undistracted by the external world. *Jyoti Mudra* can be practised at any time, but the best time is in the calm of the late evening or night. This time is ideal for turning inwards and away from the noise and distraction of the workaday routine.

CAUTION: Do not put pressure on the eyes while holding *Jyoti Mudra* — keep light and gentle pressure to avoid causing harm to this sensitive area.

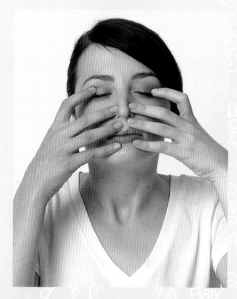

The sense openings in the face are closed in Jyoti Mudra, with the ears, eyes, nose and lips all held gently but firmly shut.

Practising Jyoti Mudra
❀

1 Sit in your choice of comfortable meditation posture (see pages 52–7) with your head, neck and spine aligned. Relax your whole body, close your eyes and bring your attention to the point between your eyebrows.

2 Inhale slowly to a mental count of ten to 12, focusing on feeling a current of *prana* rise up through your spine. As you do so, raise your arms up to your face, with your elbows parallel to the floor and pointing sideways.

3 At the end of the inhalation, hold your breath and focus on centering the *prana* you have drawn up your spine at your spiritual eye (see page 40).

4 Then place your fingers in *Jyoti Mudra* which involves closing off all the sense openings in your head: close your ears by pressing the ear flaps with your thumbs; gently hold your eyes closed by placing the index fingers on the corners of your eyelids; close your nostrils with your middle fingers; and gently squeeze your mouth shut by placing your ring fingers above the lips and your little fingers below the lips (fingertips should be touching each other).

5 While holding *Jyoti Mudra*, turn your gaze in toward the spiritual eye and feel that your fingers are directing your *prana* there. See if you can perceive its inner light and allow yourself to merge into it.

6 Holding your breath, internally repeat the mantra *Om*, directing the energy of the chant to the point between your eyebrows. See if you can see the light gathering and intensifying into a golden ring that expands to surround a sphere of deep-blue light with a silvery-white star at its centre (see box page 125).

7 Then remove your fingers and thumbs from the sense openings, keeping them gently resting on your face so that you are ready for another round.

8 Finally, exhale slowly to a mental count of ten to 12, focusing on feeling a current of *prana* descend through the spine to *muladhara chakra*.

This completes one round of *Jyoti Mudra*. Practise three rounds in total. Sit in meditative stillness, enjoying the soothing experience of this gesture.

THE SIGNIFICANCE OF OM

The sacred Sanskrit mantra *Om,* otherwise known as the Primal Sound or the Cosmic Vibration, is thought to represent the energy behind all creation. Said to contain within itself all language, letters, sounds and other mantras, its sound vibration represents union with the divine, making it the link between human consciousness and divine cosmic consciousness.

The beauty of the mantra *Om* is that it provides us with a concrete representation and experience (via sound) of what would otherwise be a difficult-to-grasp, purely abstract concept: that of the absolute, supreme reality, divine cosmic consciousness or ultimate bliss, with which we all strive to attain union. In yogic terms, this state of union is called *samadhi* and is the goal of Yoga Meditation.

The repetition (*japa;* see page 112) of *Om* is believed to produce thought waves that correspond to those of the supreme reality. So when it is chanted with faith, devotion and reverence over a sustained period of time, it encourages awareness of the presence of the divine within. As such, it is a gateway to your true divine and contented Self, a means of awakening your inner spirit and allowing you to feel more connected and at peace with yourself and the world – with an increased sense of clarity, ease and joy.

In the sacred Hindu text *Upanishad*, the mantra *Om* is described as "resplendent humming". In deep meditation this inner sound is so prominent that it drowns out all external sounds and manifests the inner sounds of the *chakras*, which are vibrating at different frequencies and therefore have different manifestations (see below). The meditation on pages 132-3 gives you the chance to experience these.

The chakra sounds as heard in meditation

MULADHARA CHAKRA – Like the humming or drone of bees. A low vibratory sound. When heard less perfectly it may sound like a motor or a drum.

SVADHISTHANA CHAKRA – Like a flute. When heard less perfectly it may sound like running water or the noise made by crickets' wings beating together.

MANIPURA CHAKRA – Like a stringed instrument such as a sitar or a harp.

ANAHATA CHAKRA – Like the flowing peal of deep bells or a gong. When heard less perfectly it sounds like tinkling bells.

VISHUDDHI CHAKRA – Like thunder or the roar of the ocean. When heard less perfectly it may sound like the wind or a waterfall.

AJNA CHAKRA (spiritual eye/medulla oblongata) – A symphony of sounds, which is *Om*, the source of all sounds.

The *Om* meditation that follows will help you to inwardly attune to the vibratory sound of divine cosmic consciousness, thus creating a sense of inner stillness and oneness with the world around you. It is particularly good to do it during the peaceful evening period, when your mind is more calm and focused.

"The sacred word Om expresses the supreme being. Constant repetition of Om and meditation on its meaning leads to samadhi."

Yoga Sutras 1:27–28

Om meditation

❦

Before you practise the *Om* meditation technique, begin with three rounds of *Maha Mudra* (see pages 114–17), a few rounds of *Nadi Shodhana* (see pages 86–7) and the *Hong Sau* technique (see pages 122–5) for 10–15 minutes, or until you feel a sense of inner calm. It is best to have been practising *Hong Sau* for at least three months in order to have settled the mind and achieved deeper levels of concentration before regularly practising this *Om* meditation.

1 Sit in your choice of comfortable meditation posture (see pages 52–7), with your head, neck and spine aligned. Place your upper arms on a suitable armrest or sit with your knees together, pulled up against your chest, and rest your elbows on your knees. Your arms and shoulders should be at a comfortable height, with no strain on your hands, arms, back or neck. When using an armrest, make sure your upper arms are resting parallel to the floor with your elbows in line with your shoulders (see page 148).

2 Raise your hands up to your head and position your fingers on your face in *Jyoti Mudra*: close your ears by gently pressing the ear flaps with your thumbs; gently close your eyes by placing your little fingers lightly on the outer corners of each eyelid; and rest your other fingers diagonally upward and inward on your forehead to direct energy toward the spiritual eye or *ajna chakra*.

3 Holding your fingers in this position, gaze with deep awareness into your spiritual eye, between your eyebrows. Then start internally chanting "Om, Om, Om", directing it at the spiritual eye, so that the mantra vibrates and resonates there. The correct pronunciation of *Om* here, the symbol of the Supreme Lord, is like the letter "o" in the alphabet but drawn out, closing with the sound "mmm". In other words, it should sound like a long, drawn-out version of the word "home" without pronouncing the "h". Equal measure should be given to both the "o" and "m" sounds.

4 As you continue to chant, simultaneously listen in your right ear for the subtle sound frequencies of your *chakras*, as the right ear is more receptive to spiritual vibrations. If you hear a distinct sound like any of those described on pages 130–131, focus your awareness totally on that. If at first you hear only your own heartbeat and breathing, then concentrate on those sounds. Over time, your mind will gradually turn inward and become calm so that you will begin to hear the more subtle sounds of the *chakras*.

5 As sensitivity develops, you are likely to hear a fainter sound behind the first one, so transfer your awareness to that. Soon, a third sound is likely to emerge behind the second, so transfer your awareness to that.

6 Continue discarding each grosser sound for the more subtle one that you hear. Your aim is to reach the source of all sound, related to your spiritual eye, or *ajna chakra* – the Primordial Vibratory Sound, *Om*. Although you are mentally chanting *Om* to keep your mind inwardly focused, it should not become a distraction from your main concentration of listening for the subtle sounds within.

7 Firstly, listen out for the *Om* sound in your right ear, later both ears, until you feel like it is coming from the centre of your brain. Then, feel it gradually descending to permeate every cell in your body and expanding outward. As your experience of this *Om* sound deepens, your consciousness expands, and you will begin to feel omnipresent, beyond the ego, mind, body and senses.

8 After listening to the inner sound vibration of *Om* for ten to 20 minutes, remain sitting for a while, enjoying the joyful stillness of your meditation and a deep sense of being at one with yourself.

ULTIMATE BLISS YOGA MEDITATION

This is the meditation to which all other Yoga Meditation practices in this book have been leading, the one in which everything comes together. The *asanas* (postures) have brought strength and steadiness so that you can sit, relaxed and still, for a long enough period of time. The purification practices have cleansed your subtle energy channels (*nadis*), helping to remove the obstacles that stop you from experiencing and realizing the divine within you. The *pranayama* (breathing techniques) have helped you gain mastery over your mind by gaining control over your vital internal energy. The meditation practices have helped to direct energy up through the *chakras* in the astral spine, calmed the mind and allowed you to experience the inner divine light within your own body.

Combined, all the practices should have helped to:

- disconnect your mind from the outward senses and the sensory objects of distraction they bring into your consciousness
- interiorize and regulate your mind and heart through self-discipline
- direct your body's vital life-force, or *prana*, up through the astral spine from the lower to the higher *chakras*
- focus your energy at the spiritual eye, or *ajna chakra*, to allow an experience of the divine inner self.

The aim of this final meditation is to raise your *prana* to the highest of the body's energy centres, known as *sahasrara chakra*, where your individual soul can truly become one with the supreme consciousness through the process of *samadhi* (divine union; see page 27) – so you can experience that lasting absolute pure joy and contentment within you, which is attained only through deep meditation.

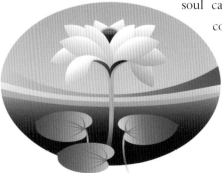

Practising Ultimate Bliss Yoga Meditation

❀

1 Sit in your choice of comfortable meditation posture (see pages 52–7), with your head, neck and spine aligned. Inhale deeply through your nose. Hold your breath and tense all the muscles in your body. Then, with a deep double exhalation through the mouth ("ha-haaa"), relax your whole body. Repeat this three times in total.

2 Remain still here, feeling the energy flowing through your body, and take a few silent moments to invoke the presence of the divine by saying something internally along the lines of: "May divine grace enliven my body, mind and spirit, and inspire, bless and guide my meditation, filling me with inner clarity, love, peace and joy."

3 Close your eyes and gently sway your spine from left to right, shifting the centre of your consciousness from the physical body and senses to your inner astral spine, imagining it like a hollow tube filled with vital, flowing energy. Once you can sense this subtle energy, stop swaying.

4 Focus your inner gaze at the midpoint between your eyebrows, at your centre of spiritual consciousness called the spiritual eye. And become aware of your breath's natural rhythm. Do not try to control it in any way, just be aware of each breath as it flows in and out. Notice where each inhalation and exhalation arises and dissolves.

5 Focus your attention on your own awareness, as if you are being attentive to attention itself. By doing so, try to become aware of the part of you that is witnessing your meditative experience – your true inner self.

6 Now breathe in deeply using *Ujjayi* breathing (see pages 98–9) to a count of ten to 15, with the air directed in the back of your throat so that it is slightly expanded to create a suction effect. (If you are not yet at ease with *Ujjayi* breathing, keep practising it, and simply breathe normally here for now.) As you inhale, be aware of a cool sensation in your throat and try to transfer that sensation up your astral spine to the medulla oblongata and across to your spiritual eye.

7 Hold your breath here for the count of three internal *Om* chants.

8 Next, exhale slowly and deeply with *Ujjayi* breathing (if you are familiar with it) to a count of ten to 15, being aware of the warm sensation of the breath as it moves down through the spine from your eyebrow centre to the base of your spine.

9 Then, without a pause, begin to inhale up your spine again. Practise 12 cycles of this deep breathing up and down your spine until you feel your spine vibrating and pulsating with energy.

10 Then allow your breathing to return to its normal pattern and just be aware of your energy moving up and down, deep within your spine. Follow the movement of your breath and listen carefully to the inner sound it makes.

11 As you breathe in and the energy moves up your spine, internally repeat *Hong*. As you breathe out and the energy moves down your spine, internally repeat *Sau*.

12 With attentive focus listen to the *Hong* on each inhalation and the *Sau* on each exhalation. Merge your attention with the flow of breath and identify yourself more and more with the vibration of the mantra. To do this, try to visualize the *Hong Sau* mantra as light or energy and feel yourself immersed in it until you feel you have become one with it and are blessed by it.

13 Mentally affirm: "I am spirit, I am pure I-awareness, the ever-Existing, ever-conscious, ever-blissful Self."

14 Then remain in the blissful stillness of the meditative space you have created for as long as you naturally can, enjoying the expansion of consciousness and sense of oneness with the divine.

15 When you are ready, return to normal breathing and gradually become aware of the sensations in your physical body. Then place your hands together in prayer position in front of your heart and offer thanks to the source of the divine within you – for grace, blessings, energy and power.

16 Chant *Om Shanti* (a mantra for peace) three times to send peace and love to all beings in the universe. Let every breath that flows from you create a strong current of divine service to all beings.

17 Slowly open your eyes, then remain quietly seated for a short while to enjoy the sense of peace from your meditation. Allow this inner calm and contentedness to permeate into your everyday consciousness.

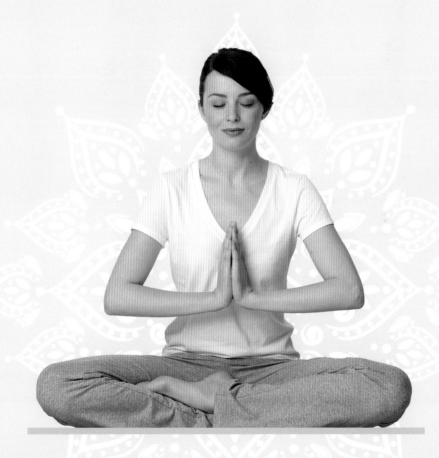

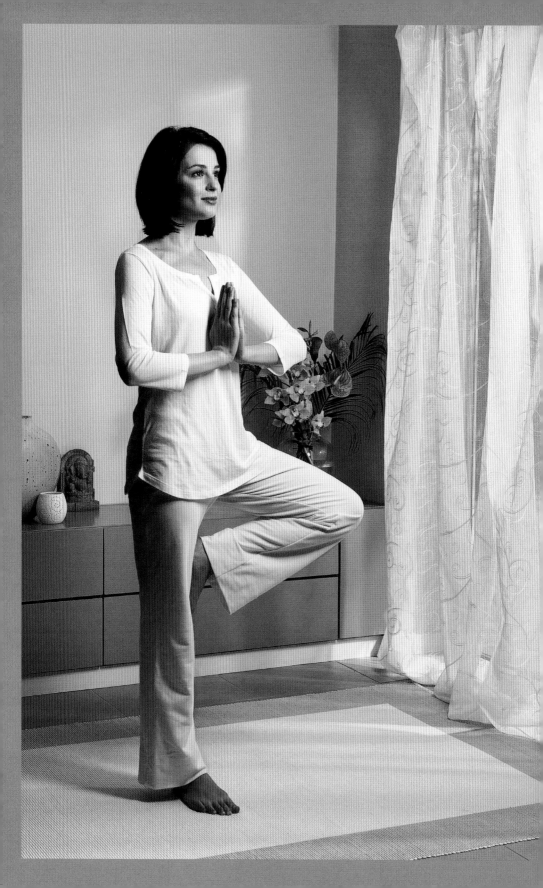

CHAPTER 8

DEVELOPING YOUR PRACTICE

INTEGRATING YOUR YOGA MEDITATION INTO DAILY LIVING

This chapter is where you learn how to put all the Yoga Meditation practices in this book together in the form of routines of different lengths – with five choices for both the morning and the evening – depending on your individual requirements.

Although in our busy lives we often don't have as much time as we might like to practise yoga and meditation, there is usually a way to fit in at least 15 minutes of practice a day, whether that means getting up 15 minutes earlier or going to bed 15 minutes later. The shortest of the routines in the pages that follow is therefore 15 minutes long, while the longest, most beneficial one is 1 hour 45 minutes long. The more regularly you can commit to one or more of these routines, the greater sense of inner peace, contentment and connectedness you are likely to experience in daily life.

In order to obtain optimum benefits from your Yoga Meditation, it is, however, essential that you lead a lifestyle that is fully supportive of your goals off the yoga mat as well as on it. Guidance is therefore given on a healthy overall, daily routine, including what time to get up and go to bed, an optimal cleansing routine and the ideal diet.

LIVING WITH AWARENESS

In order to really get the most from the Yoga Meditation practices in this book, it is important to maintain a balanced all-round lifestyle to complement them. Commitment to optimum health requires not only sufficient exercise and dedication to a spiritual practice such as Yoga Meditation, but also wholesome nutrition, adequate relaxation and sufficient sleep.

In yogic terms, it is important to keep the body and mind healthy not only in order to feel physically fit but also so that they remain fit vehicles through which the true divine inner Self can express itself, allowing you to experience a sense of oneness and harmony in life.

The following daily guidelines will help you to maintain a healthy and balanced body and mind to this end. Although it may not always be possible to follow all the guidelines within the restraints of busy, modern life, any that you do follow will be of enormous benefit.

Rise early

According to yogic thinking, the early morning (before 6 am) is filled with *prana*, making this the best period to get up in the morning and also the most rewarding time to meditate.

The period between 4 and 6 am is believed to be when lightness and clarity predominate, and your mind and body have maximum chance for feeling fresh. Sleeping beyond 6 am, on the other hand, is likely to make us feel more sluggish, tired and experience slow movement of the bowels.

Empty your bladder and bowels

It is important as soon as you get up in the morning to go to the toilet and get your bladder and bowels moving. If a bowel movement does not come easily, try drinking a mug of hot water with half a fresh lemon squeezed into it, a pinch of salt and a teaspoon of honey. Then drink another mug of plain warm water. The lemon and salt have a cleansing, drawing-out effect, and the honey is a tonic for the colon.

Clean your teeth and tongue, and gargle

It is important to regularly remove toxins and bacteria from your body. So at least twice a day, use a small or medium soft-bristled toothbrush to carefully brush your teeth. Ayurveda, Indian traditional medicine, recommends a toothpaste with astringent, bitter and pungent flavours, such as myrrh, propolis, neem or peppermint. A toothpaste that contains baking soda is also good. Once you have brushed your teeth, also floss between them to dislodge any bacteria. It is also recommended that you gently scrape your tongue with a tongue scraper or the edge of a teaspoon to remove the bacterial coating and to dispel bad breath. Finally, gargle with a little warm water to clear and soothe your throat.

Rinse your nose

It is good yogic practice to regularly use what is called a *neti* pot (similar to a small teapot, but with a special spout) to rinse out your nasal passages. To do so, fill the pot with warm water and dissolve one teaspoon of salt in it. Leaning over a washbasin, tilt your head to the left side and placing the spout

Digestive remedy

❀

If you suffer from constipation, bloating, flatulence or indigestion, you can try drinking *triphala* (available to buy from reputable herbal suppliers) – an Ayurvedic powder remedy blended from three fruits: *haritaki, bibhitaki* and *amalaki*. Dissolve one teaspoonful of *triphala* powder in a mug of hot water, then let it stand for a few minutes before drinking. It is best taken in the evening, half an hour before sleep.

slightly in the right nostril, slowly pour the water up your nose so that it flows out of the left nostril. The warm salty water flushes out mucus and dust, cleansing the lining of the nostrils. To expel the excess of water from your nostrils, breathe in and out rapidly through the nose.

Give your body a massage

Ayurveda recommends daily massage, if possible, before a bath, to encourage the release of waste products from the body. Massaging the skin stimulates blood circulation and encourages the flow of lymph. It also cleanses, nourishes, relaxes and rejuvenates the body.

- Warm some sesame oil (organic, cold-pressed, and less than six months old). If it irritates your skin, use coconut oil or sweet almond oil instead.
- Sit on a bath towel and apply the warm oil all over your body from head to foot, taking about ten minutes to do so. Use up and down or circular movements of your hands to smooth the oil into your skin.
- Then relax for five minutes to allow your skin to absorb the oil.
- If you are pressed for time, a two- or three-minute massage is still useful, focusing mainly on your head and feet.

Take a warm bath or shower

After your oil massage, take a warm bath or shower using a mild soap to cleanse the oil from your skin.

Follow your *sadhana*

Sadhana is a Sanskrit word meaning "spiritual" practice. Having thoroughly cleansed your body, you can now put on clean, comfortable clothes and begin your Yoga Meditation *sadhana* from this book (see pages 146–53 for options of sessions of varying lengths, combining the practices in the book). It is important to be regular in your daily *sadhana*, as its purpose is for you to discover your true joyful inner Self and to feel at peace with the world.

Eat a healthy breakfast

Eat a nourishing light breakfast such as fresh fruit of your choice, muesli with a few soaked and peeled almonds, porridge of oats, millet or buckwheat flakes, or buckwheat pancakes, alongside a cup of herbal tea, in a calm, pleasant atmosphere – in silence if possible.

Make lunch the main meal of the day

What is known in yogic terms as the "digestive fire" is at its strongest and most efficient at midday. Eat in a relaxed atmosphere – in silence if possible. Chew your food well. And do not dilute your digestive juices by drinking glasses of water or juice while eating; instead, allow half an hour after food before drinking. Sit quietly for five minutes, then take a short walk of up to 15 minutes if you can to aid digestion. Then resume your afternoon activities. The hours between 2 and 6 pm are optimal for mental activities.

Have a light evening meal

After any evening Yoga Meditation practice, have a light dinner, ensuring that you have left at least three hours since lunch for adequate digestion. It is best to avoid yogurt, animal protein and raw ingredients at this time as they are hard to digest. Do not read or watch television while you eat. And try to eat only three-quarters of your capacity; stop when you are comfortably full.

Bedtime

Yoga agrees with the maxim "early to bed early to rise, makes a person healthy, wealthy and wise". To ensure you get a full night of deep rest, which is vital for optimum health, go to bed no later than 10 pm. Between 10 pm and 2 am is believed to be an active period of the night, so if you are awake then, it will make you feel lively, alert and unlikely to have a good night's rest. Staying up late may also contribute to insomnia, digestive and elimination problems, high blood pressure and poor concentration.

MAKING YOGA MEDITATION
A DAILY REALITY

For all-round development of both your mind and body, and to awaken and harness your physical and mental energy, it is best to practise Yoga Meditation twice a day if at all possible – once when you get up in the morning to start the day off well and again in the evening to help you unwind – even if it is only 15 minutes each time. Alternatively, if you have more time either in the morning or evening, you could opt for a longer practice then.

The selection of timed Morning and Evening Routines that follows has been specially created from the many invaluable practices explained throughout this book. Choose which of the five timed routines (15 minutes, 30 minutes, 1 hour, 1 hour 15 minutes, or 1 hour 45 minutes) best suits you depending on how much time you have and which practices you are comfortable with at this stage on your Yoga Meditation journey. Remember to reassess your timing needs every now and then in order to get the most from your practice.

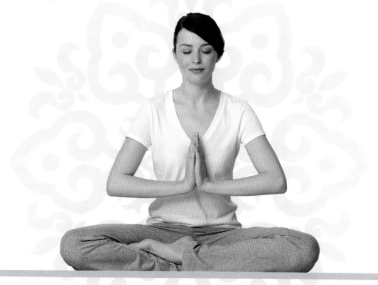

Practice and time

❀

The routines that follow are flexible, so if you sense that it is beneficial to give more attention to certain techniques, then by all means do so. But always try to give as much time as you can to the meditation practices (for example, at the weekend you might have time to do longer meditations), as experiencing stillness, peace and a sense of connectedness in meditation is ultimately the aim of all the practices.

Please bear in mind that the timings given are approximate, based on how long it takes an average practitioner to do them. However, every individual works at their own pace so do leave some flexibility around the suggested timings, especially if you are new to yoga and meditation. Do not feel worried if some practices take more or less time to do. Note also that any discrepancy between the length of time suggested for a practice in the following routines and given in the main entry for that practice is because the timings here have been amended to work within each routine's timed framework.

❀

In the Spirit of Meditation

More important than when and where you meditate, or what techniques you use, are your attitude and the spirit of the heart in which you practise, and your self-discipline and regularity in practising meditation. Through regular, disciplined practice you will develop your awareness, wisdom, energy and joy to a level that you can skilfully integrate your experience of centred inner calm, peace and joy into your everyday life.

MORNING ROUTINES

The morning routines on the right will awaken the energy within you, giving you the vitality you need to start the day. The combination of recommended practices within each routine will encourage free circulation of vital forces, stimulating your glands, improving blood and lymph circulation, and releasing body wastes as well as any mental-emotional tensions and blockages. The result of doing these routines regularly will be increased energy, enhanced clarity and a calmer mind.

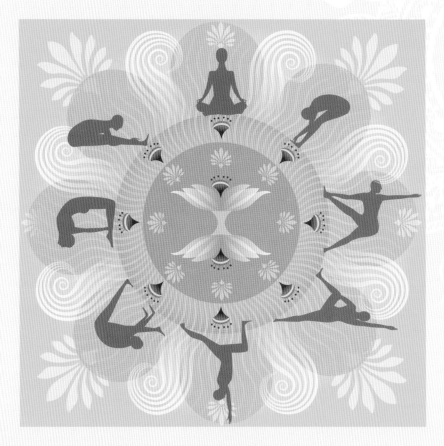

15-MINUTE ROUTINE

1 Purification practices
   - *Nadi Shodhana*
     3 minutes; see pages 86–7
   - *Agnisara Kriya*
     2 minutes; see pages 88–9

2 Meditation practices
   - *Hong Sau*
     10 minutes; see pages 122–5

30-MINUTE ROUTINE

1 *Asana* Practices
   - Warming up
     5 minutes; see pages 64–7
   - Sun Salutation Sequence
     10 minutes; see pages 68–71

2 Meditation Practices
   - *Maha Mudra*
     5 minutes; see pages 114–17
   - *Hong Sau*
     10 minutes; see pages 122–5

1-HOUR ROUTINE

1 *Asana* practices
   - Warming up
     5 minutes; see pages 64–7
   - Energizing Morning Sequence
     10 minutes; see pages 72–5

2 Purification practices
   - *Nadi Shodhana*
     5 minutes; see pages 86–7

3 *Pranayama* practices
   - Complete Yogic Breath
     5 minutes; see pages 96–7
   - *Bhastrika Pranayama*
     5 minutes; see pages 100–101

4 Meditation practices
   - *Maha Mudra*
     5 minutes; see pages 114–17
   - *Hong Sau*
     10 minutes; see pages 122–5
   - *Navi Kriya*
     5 minutes; see pages 126–7
   - *Om* Meditation
     10 minutes; see pages 132–3

1 HOUR 15 MINUTE ROUTINE

1 *Asana* practices
   - Warming up
     5 minutes; see pages 64–7
   - Sun Salutation Sequence:
     10 minutes; see pages 68–71 .

2 Purification Practices
   - *Nadi Shodhana*
     5 minutes; see pages 86–7
   - *Agnisara Kriya*
     3 minutes; see pages 88–9
   - *Kapalabhati*
     5 minutes; see page 92
   - *Ashvini Mudra*
     2 minutes; see page 93

3 Meditation practices
   - *Maha Mudra*
     5 minutes; see pages 114–17
   - *Hong Sau*
     15 minutes; see pages 122–5
   - *Navi Kriya*
     5 minutes; see pages 126–7
   - *Om* Meditation
     20 minutes; see pages 132–3

1 HOUR 45 MINUTE ROUTINE

1 *Asana* practices
  • Warming up
    5 minutes; see pages 64–7
  • Sun Salutation Sequence
    10 minutes; see pages 68–71
  • Energizing Morning Sequence
    10 minutes; see pages 72–5

2 Purification practices
  • *Nadi Shodhana*
    5 minutes; see pages 86–7
  • *Agnisara Kriya*
    3 minutes; see pages 88–9
  • *Kapalabhati*
    5 minutes; see page 92
  • *Ashvini Mudra*
    2 minutes; see page 93

3 *Pranayama* practices
  • Complete Yogic Breath
    5 minutes; see pages 96–97
  • *Bhastrika Pranayama*
    5 minutes; see pages 100–101
  • *Bhramari Pranayama*
    5 minutes; see page 102–3
  • *Kundalini Pranayama*
    5 minutes; see pages 104–5

4 Meditation practices
  • *Maha Mudra*
    5 minutes; see pages 114–17
  • *Bija* mantras
    5 minutes; see pages 118–19
  • *Hong Sau*
    10 minutes; see pages 122–5
  • *Navi Kriya*
    5 minutes; see page 126–7
  • *Om* Meditation
    20 minutes; see pages 132–3

"Be calmly active, and actively calm. That is the way of a yogi. Meditate regularly, and you will find a joy inside that is real."

Paramhansa Yogananda

EVENING ROUTINES

The evening routines that follow focus mainly on practices that have a relaxing effect on your mind and body at the end of a busy day. If you are doing a routine that involves *asana* and *pranayama* practices, it is best to do it just after work, whereas a meditation-based routine is more suitable for just before bedtime to ensure a good night's sleep.

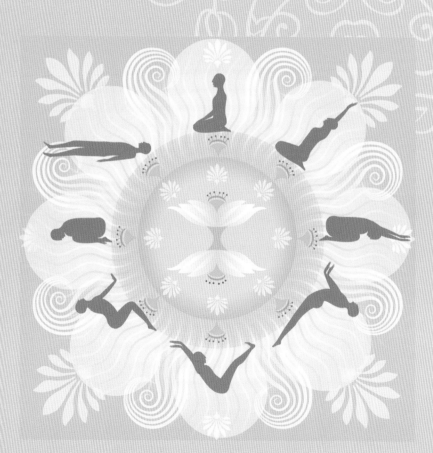

15-MINUTE ROUTINE

1 Meditation practices
  - *Maha Mudra*
    5 minutes; see pages 114–17

  - *Hong Sau*
    10 minutes; see pages 122–5

30-MINUTE ROUTINE

1 Meditation practices
  - *Maha Mudra*
    5 minutes; see pages 114–17
  - *Hong Sau*
    10 minutes; see pages 122–5

  - Ultimate Bliss Yoga Meditation
    15 minutes; see pages 134–7

1-HOUR ROUTINE

1 Meditation practices
  - *Maha Mudra*
    5 minutes; see pages 114–17
  - *Hong Sau*
    10 minutes; see pages 122–5

  - *Jyoti Mudra*
    5 minutes; see pages 128–9
  - *Om* Meditation
    10 minutes; see pages 132–3
  - Ultimate Bliss Yoga Meditation
    30 minutes; see pages 134–7

1 HOUR 15 MINUTE ROUTINE

1 *Asana* practices
- Warming up
  5 minutes; see pages 64–7
- Relaxing Evening Sequence
  10 minutes; see page 76–9

2 Purification practices
- *Nadi Shodhana*
  5 minutes; see pages 86–7

3 *Pranayama* practices
- *Ujjayi Pranayama*
  5 minutes; see pages 98–9

4 Meditation practices
- Steady gazing
  5 minutes; see page 113
- *Maha Mudra*
  5 minutes; see pages 114–17
- *Hong Sau*
  10 minutes; see pages 122–5
- *Jyoti Mudra*
  5 minutes; see pages 128–9
- *Om* Meditation
  10 minutes; see pages 132–3
- Ultimate Bliss Yoga Meditation
  15 minutes; see pages 134–7

❀

Mastering the art of meditation

It is important to remember that meditation requires dedication and discipline, so do not give up on it before you have given it a proper chance. If you find it difficult to sit in stillness, the trick is simply to set aside more time for each meditation session. By being willing to sit for a longer period of time, you will allow your thoughts more time to slow and settle down. As most experienced meditators will tell you, true meditative stillness usually occurs after between 45 minutes and an hour. To reach this state, you will need to persist with a steady effort. If you feel a resistance to sitting, simply try to let go of the thoughts that are holding you back and bring your attention and awareness back to your breath or the mantra *Om*.

1 HOUR 45 MINUTE ROUTINE

1 *Asana* practices
   • **Warming up**
     5 mins; see pages 64–7
   • **Relaxing Evening Sequence**
     10 minutes; see pages 76–9
   • **Cool Down Sequence**
     10 minutes; see pages 80–83

2 **Purification practices**
   • *Nadi Shodhana*
     5 minutes; see pages 86–7

3 *Pranayama* practices
   • *Ujjayi Pranayama*
     5 minutes; see pages 98–9
   • *Bhramari Pranayama*
     5 minutes; see pages 102–3

4 Meditation practices
   • *Maha Mudra*
     5 minutes; see pages 114–17
   • *Bija* mantras
     10 minutes; see pages 118–19
   • *Hum* mantra
     5 minutes; see pages 120–21
   • *Hong Sau*
     10 minutes; see pages 122–5
   • *Om* Meditation
     15 minutes; see pages 132–3
   • **Ultimate Bliss Yoga Meditation**
     20 minutes; see pages 134–7

FURTHER READING

- Ashley-Farrand, Thomas, *Chakra Mantras*, Weiser Books, San Francisco, 2006

- Avalon, Arthur, *The Serpent Power*, Dover Publications, new York, 1974

- Bryant, Edwin F, *The Yoga Sutras of Patanjali*, North Point Press, New York, 2009

- The Dalai Lama, *Beyond Religion*, Rider, London, 2012

- Davis, Roy Eugene, *The Science of Self-Realization*, CSA Press, Lakemont, Georgia, 2004

- Davis, Roy Eugene, *Paramhansa Yogananda As I Knew Him*, CSA Press, Lakemont, Georgia, 2005

- Davis, Roy Eugene, *Seven Lessons in Conscious Living*, CSA Press, Lakemont, Georgia, 2013

- Feuerstein, Georg, *The Deeper Dimensions of Yoga*, Shambhala Publications, Boston, 2003

- Iyengar, B.K.S, *Core of the Yoga Sutras*, HarperThorsons, London, 2012

- Kriyananda, Swami, *The Essence of Self-Realization*, Crystal Clarity Publishers, Nevada City, 1990

- Kriyananda, Swami, *God is for Everyone*, Crystal Clarity Publishers, Nevada City, 2003

- Kriyananda, Swami, *The Essence of the Bhagavad Gita*, Crystal Clarity Publishers, Nevada City, 2006

- Kriyananda, Swami, *Paramhansa Yogananda - A Biography*, Crystal Clarity Publishers, Nevada City, 2011

- Mehta, Mira, *Yoga Explained*, Angus Books, London, 2004

- Niranjanananda, Swami, *Prana, Pranayama, Prana Vidya,* Yoga Publications Trust, Bihar, 1994

- Selbie and Steinmetz, *The Yugas*, Crystal Clarity Publishers, Nevada City, 2010

- Stephens, Mark, *Yoga Sequencing*, North Atlantic Books, Berkeley, California, 2012

- Sturgess, Stephen, *The Yoga Book*, Watkins Publishing, London, 2002

- Sturgess, Stephen, *The Book of Chakras and Subtle Bodies*, Watkins Publishing, London, 2013

- Vishnu-Devananda, Swami, *Hatha Yoga Pradipika*, Lotus Publishing, New York, 1987

- Yogananda, Paramhansa, *Where There is Light*, Self-Realization Fellowship, Los Angeles, 1989

- Yogananda, Paramhansa, *Autobiography of A Yogi*, Crystal Clarity Publishers Nevada City, 1994

- Yogananda, Paramhansa, *Journey to Self-Realization*, Self-Realization Fellowship, Los Angeles, 1997

- Yogananda, Paramhansa, *Metaphysical Meditations*, Self-Realization Fellowship, Los Angeles, 1998

- Yogananda, Paramhansa, In the Sanctuary of the Soul, Self-Realization Fellowship, Los Angeles, 1998

- Yogananda, Paramhansa, Inner Peace, Self-Realization Fellowship, Los Angeles, 1999

- Yogananda, Paramhansa, God Talks with Arjuna - The Bhagavad Gita, Self-Realization Fellowship, Los Angeles, 2002

- Yogananda, Paramhansa, How to be Happy all the Time, Crystal Clarity Publishers Nevada City, 2006

- Yogananda, Paramhansa, How to be a Success, Crystal Clarity Publishers, Nevada City, 2008

- Yukteswar, Swami Sri, The Holy Science, Self-Realization Fellowship, Los Angeles, 1997

FURTHER RESOURCES

For further information on the Kriya Yoga teachings of Stephen Sturgess in London visit: www.yogananda-kriyayoga.org.uk or email stephensturgess@hotmail.com

For further information on Kriya Yoga meditation in general:

UK:
www.kriyayogacentre.org.uk
www.srf-london.org.uk

USA:
www.ananda.org
www.expandinglight.org
www.csa-davis.org
www.yogananda-srf.org

INDIA:
www.anandaindia.org

ITALY:
www.ananda.it

INDEX

ACKNOWLEDGMENTS

Many thanks to Bob Saxton, who initially got the project off the ground. To Kelly Thompson, the managing editor who paid meticulous attention to detail, while keeping always warm-hearted and cheerful; and to Tania Ahsan who also cheerfully worked on the editing. To Luana Gobbo, the graphic designer, who made a lovely design of the book. To Jules Selmes, the photographer, and his assistant Adam, both of whom worked hard to get those beautiful shots of the model. And to the model herself, Tess Dimas (MOT), who looked naturally calm and serene. And finally, a big thank you to the Christiane Beauregard, the illustrator who contributed the beautiful and colourful illustrations to the book.